FREED TO LEAD

F3 and the Unshackling
of the Modern-day Warrior

by
Dredd and OBT

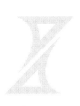

FREED TO LEAD
F3 and the Unshackling of the Modern-day Warrior

Copyright © 2014 by The Iron Project, LLC

All Rights Reserved.

No part of this publication may be reproduced in any form
or by any means, including photocopying, scanning, recording, or otherwise
without prior written permission of the copyright holder.
Cover illustration based on Joe Rosenthal photograph of U.S. Marines
of the 28th Regiment, 5th Division, raising the American flag atop Mt. Suribachi, Iwo
Jima, on Feb. 23, 1945. Used with permission
of The Associated Press.

Interior illustrations by Jason Hendrickson.

Cover and interior design by Benard Owuondo and Lazar Kackarovski.

ISBN: 978-0-9912381-0-1

TABLE OF CONTENTS

PROLOGUE   *7*

PART ONE: Solving a Problem
We Didn't Know Existed   *9*
Chapter 1: *The Explanation*   *10*
Chapter 2: *Why We Are Here*   *14*
Chapter 3: *Forty-three Feet of Good Road*   *21*
Chapter 4: *Half the Mission*   *24*

PART TWO: The Problem   *35*
Chapter 1: *A Good Place to Stop*   *36*
Chapter 2: *SadClown Syndrome*   *39*
Chapter 3: *Bowling Ball Grip*   *42*
Chapter 4: *Pogo40*   *44*
Chapter 5: *The Sifter*   *49*
Chapter 6: *The Reacher*   *57*

PART THREE: The Solution   *63*
Chapter 1: *The Full Mission*   *64*
Chapter 2: *The Magnet of the First F*   *67*
ShovelFlags and BackBlasts   68

Time, Place, and Manner *72*
The Starfish *76*
I2 *79*
Mean Mean Stride *82*
The Museum of Failure *86*
HTC *93*

Chapter 3: The Glue of the Second F 96
Regions and Nomads *96*
The Coffeeteria, the HDHH, and the Convergence *100*
CSAUP *101*
The Magical Glue of CSAUP *104*

Chapter 4: The Dynamite of the Third F 108
Living Third *110*
The Reverse-Flow Incubator *114*
Concentrica *119*
D2X *122*
   The Dolphin 123
   The Daffodil 124
Putting it Together *129*
Purpose *130*
The Third 500 *136*
Locked Shields of the Minivan Centurions *143*

ACKNOWLEDGMENTS *146*

ABOUT THE AUTHORS *148*

DEDICATION

To the 34 men who posted on the foggy morning of 1/1/11 at Alexander Graham Middle School for the first workout of what would become F3. And to our own Ms and the Ms across F3 Nation; they tolerate what we do, and they are the ones for whom we do it.

PROLOGUE

THIS BOOK IS THE story behind the success of F3, the network of small, free workout groups for men that we launched on January 1st, 2011, with a single New Year's Day workout at a Charlotte, North Carolina, middle school. As of this writing (late 2013) there are 220+ scheduled weekly F3 workouts — primarily in the Carolinas, but also in locations as far-flung as Cleveland, Ohio, Denver, Colorado, and Washington, D.C. Each week, more than 1,500 men participate in an F3 workout and, all told, more than 2,500 men have experienced an F3 workout.

The defining characteristics of an F3 workout are that it takes place outdoors, almost always at an unpleasantly early hour; that it is led by one of the participants (not a paid fitness instructor); and that it is physically challenging while being inclusive of all men who show up for the workout.

No one has ever been turned away from an F3 workout; no one has ever been charged for an F3 workout.

F3's growth has outpaced even our wildest 1/1/11 dreams, but that's not the story we're here to tell. What we think makes this a story worth spending your hard-earned cash to read is F3's impact on the lives of the men who participate in it.

In the pages ahead, we will explain how we came to realize – well after F3 had become a sort of runaway train – that it solved a

Problem (perhaps THE Problem) that plagued many of the men we knew (something we call SadClown Syndrome).

Part One of this book gives a high-level overview of the three Fs in our name (Fitness, Fellowship and Faith). We'll take a quick look at how an F3 workout runs, the broad organizing principles of F3 and why those formats seem to work particularly well (in the process, we'll throw a lot of F3 Lingo at you – look for explanations in the sidebars).

Part Two really digs into the Problem, as we've come to understand it through our F3 experience and our own lives.

Part Three returns to F3 in much deeper detail. We break down each of the three Fs (Fitness, Fellowship, and Faith) and explain how each exists within the F3 framework and how the F3 approach to each one helps address a different aspect of the Problem.

We've written this book for one reason and one reason only: to get our Solution to the Problem in front of more men. It's the same reason we started F3 in the first place. So read the book, pass it along – and use it to Do Something.

PART 1

SOLVING A PROBLEM WE DIDN'T KNOW EXISTED

1

THE EXPLANATION

F3 IS A SOLUTION to a problem, THE Problem (we believe). We didn't invent F3 to solve the Problem. We couldn't have done that because when F3 was born, we didn't yet know how to define or even to describe the Problem. What we knew, what we felt, was that something was wrong in our lives as men. Something was off. Despite all we had — our families, our houses, our careers — despite all these great things we had, we were still missing something. This feeling we had was the effect of the Problem on a man's life.

This feeling is very difficult to describe. It was as if we had packed very carefully for a business trip but knew as we drove to the airport that the one thing necessary for its success had been left out of the suitcase. We didn't know what that left-behind thing was or why its omission would cause the trip to fail. We just knew we didn't have it, and we were getting on the plane without it anyway because life gave us no choice. Eventually the plane would land, we would open up that suitcase, and we would finally discover what that needful thing was. Only then it would be too late.

It was a frustrating and helpless feeling. Even without being able to describe this missing thing, we discovered that F3 somehow provided it. It helped dissipate that helpless feeling by filling a hole in our lives, even though we couldn't put our finger on exactly where the hole was.

If it sounds like the prescription preceded the diagnosis, that is because it was the way it worked for us. And because it did work, we didn't (initially) spend a lot of time worrying about or defining the Problem that F3 was solving for us. Once it helped us, we wanted to see it help other men who seemed to be suffering from the same amorphous ailment. That's how this all started. A couple of lucky beggars trying to show the other starving men where and how they had found a crumb.

To do that, to share the solution we had stumbled upon, we had to do a lot of explaining. Men had questions they wanted answered before they would try something this radical. At first, we were not very good at explaining. There was no real context for what we were saying. We sounded like Eskimos trying to describe the qualities of an igloo to men who have lived their lives in a rain forest.

But (like anything else) the more we gave the Explanation, the better we got at it. We learned from our mistakes. The questions men asked us started to fall into a recognizable pattern that we could anticipate. That gave us confidence. We convinced a few men to join us. Before long, some of those men we convinced wanted to share it too. So, we started teaching them how to give the Explanation so they wouldn't repeat our earlier mistakes.

At first, there were several problems with our teaching approach. We were inconsistent. We didn't define our terms very well. We hadn't even come up with the name "F3," so men were trying to learn how to explain something without a name.

But we trudged on, despite our initial ineptitude. We learned from our mistakes and persisted in our efforts to improve, as the men who accepted our Explanation persisted in their desire to know how to give it themselves. Eventually, we started doing it well enough that the men we were teaching began asking us to write the Explanation down so they could refer to it later and give it to the men they were trying to help.

That was a reasonable request. But we resisted it, for three reasons. First, the Explanation was dynamic. As F3 grew and changed, the Explanation grew and changed.

Second, we didn't want to write something down that was incomplete. And writing the Explanation would be difficult. We're not authors. It was one thing to talk and another to write. Maybe it would be so hard that we would fail, after wasting a lot of time trying. We didn't want to fail, and we didn't want to waste time. Finally, whether we succeeded or failed at writing the Explanation, we didn't think we had the time to do it. We had jobs, families, planes to catch, and bills to pay. We were already spending huge amounts of time growing F3 and giving/teaching the Explanation. Where were we going to find the additional time it would take to record what we were doing as we did it? Bottom Line: we didn't translate (or commit) the Explanation to written form, not for a long time.

We kept giving/teaching the Explanation face to face, to one man (or small groups of men) at a time. It was inefficient, but it seemed to work, and we liked doing it that way. It was a mission. When men asked us when we were going to write the Explanation we would say, "Someday, we're working on it." But we weren't. We were procrastinating.

That might have been where the story ended, if F3 had not begun to spread to other cities. Those men needed the Explanation as well, but it was too far to drive to teach them face-to-face. We tried the telephone. We tried e-mail. There are pieces of the Explanation on the F3Nation website, but it was disjointed and didn't hang together. None of these half-measures succeeded in providing the Explanation in an integrated form to men whom we could not physically reach.

Finally, we admitted to ourselves that distance so degraded the quality of the Explanation that it wasn't serving these men at all. We were failing in our mission. We accepted that we would have to either invest the time required to write the Explanation (and take the risk that we would fail in the effort), or tell the men in distant cities that we weren't willing to do what it would take to help them. Once we had admitted that truth to ourselves, the decision wasn't difficult. We chose to write.

WHY WE ARE HERE

THE OBVIOUS AND LOGICAL way to write the Explanation would be to start with the Problem itself. However, from the many hours we have spent giving the Explanation verbally, we know that wouldn't work. To understand F3, the prescription has to precede the diagnosis.

In brief: F3 is a network of men's small workout groups that is built around three "Fs": Fitness, Fellowship, and Faith.

The Fitness F (the "First F") consists primarily of the Workout. There are a few (but only a few) rules about the Workout:

1. It must be free of charge;
2. It must be open to all men;
3. It must be held outdoors, rain or shine, heat or cold;
4. It must be led in a rotating fashion by men who participate in the Workout, with no training or certification necessary; and
5. It must end with a Circle of Trust (the "COT").

The F3 Lexicon

We will be calling periodic timeouts to give you these sidebar explanations of some of the inside lingo we use in F3. It's good prep for going on our website the first time – otherwise the Workout writeups (BackBlasts) are liable to make your head spin. So here goes.

Circle of Trust (COT): *The gathering of F3 men at the end of each Workout for purposes of generating a count, sharing names, making announcements and saying a quick prayer of thanks.*

Q: *This is the designation given to the Workout leader.*

Post: *To show up for a Workout*

The PAX: *The men who post for a given Workout*

Mothership: *The first F3 Workout, held Saturdays at 7 a.m. at Alexander Graham Middle School in Charlotte, N.C.*

FNG: *Stands for "Friendly New Guy" – placeholder for an F3 newbie who has yet to be given his F3 nickname.*

F3 Name: *Nickname given to a man upon successful completion of his first F3 Workout. The Workout Q has nicknaming privileges.*

Splashing Merlot: *Throwing up during an F3 Workout.*

Emotional Headlock (EH): *The process of talking a guy into posting for his first F3 Workout.—i.e., "I must have put him in the Emotional Headlock five or six times before he finally posted."*

Sponsor: *The person who EHs an FNG; it's generally considered good Sponsor form to accompany your FNG to his first Workout.*

Six: *Code for your "sixth point of contact with the earth" – i.e., your butt. Used both to refer to your rear end and to the last man in an F3 Workout group, i.e., "Is the Six here? Can we start the COT?"*

These rules, which we call our Core Principles, are simple and (with the exception of the COT, which we will describe in Part Three, Chapter Four) self-explanatory. Other than these principles, F3 has no rules, just a lot of suggestions. The Q is free to design and run the Workout as he sees fit. The Q gets feedback from the PAX about whether his leadership is any good. Feedback is generally immediate, abundant, and forthcoming, whether the Q wants it or not.

We started the Mothership on Saturday, January 1st, 2011. In the three years since that day, the Mothership has spawned many other Workouts, both on Saturday and on every other day of the week. Every Workout takes on the unique characteristics of the Qs who originally plant it and the Qs who eventually run it (not always the same men). F3 members are free to Post to any Workout they want, so there is a lot of competition among the Qs over who runs the best Workout. "Best" usually means hardest. Make it hard, and they will come.

When a man Posts to a Workout for the first time he is a Friendly New Guy. A man is only an FNG at the very beginning of his first Workout. At the end of the workout, at the COT, the Q gives the FNG his F3 Name, a nickname he will go by ever afterwards among the PAX.

F3 Names

F3 nicknames generally fall into three categories (which often blur into each other): Quick & Dirty, Insulting, and Obscurely Referential. The best nicknames are all three at once. Here are a few of our favorites.

Belk: *Given to a guy whose last name is Dillard – Belk and Dillard's are rival Charlotte department store chains.*

Five-0: *This guy's last name is Lay, which sounds like "lei," which gets you to Hawaii and the TV show Hawaii Five-0.*

Egypt: *Given to a guy whose last name is Boehmfolk (drop the "l" from "folk" and you'll get the idea...)*

FaSoLa: *Matt's dad is Karl Doerre (pronounced "doh-RAY") so Karl was nicknamed DoReMi. When Matt posted for the first time, the tradition had to continue, so he became FSL.*

Once named, the man is a member of F3. There is no other initiation required. There is no fee. F3 has no registration form. All a man has to do is Post, make it through to the COT, and accept his F3 Name. That's it.

Solving a Problem We Didn't Know Existed

PART 1

The "I Have To Get In Shape" Excuse

Probably the most common excuse we get from guys about why they can't/won't come out to an F3 workout is "I have to get in shape before I come out to work out with you guys. Which, as Dredd likes to say, is a little like a guy telling you he has to get drunk before he can come meet you out at the local bar for a few beers.

From the start, F3 workouts have been designed to accommodate guys at a wide range of fitness levels in a format that allows everyone to get a good workout while staying together as a group. We often remind FNGs that "it's you against you" out there (i.e., not you against that 25-year-old who just a couple years ago was playing D1 soccer for an ACC school) and we've found that to work remarkably well to get guys in and working out. Next thing they know, five or six weeks have passed and they're moving up the ladder and no longer at the back of the pack.

We also used to think that there were some guys that F3 couldn't help – guys who were too overweight or too far removed from physical activity. Then guys within F3 started taking it on themselves to start CORE workouts (for guys unable or unready to do much running) and a "Silver Bullet Express" workout for guys who are guys who are over 60. So now, we just say that the only guys F3 can help are guys with a Y chromosome.

There are a variety of ways an FNG can find his way to his first Post. One FNG read about F3 in the local newspaper and showed up the next day (we named him FishWrap). Most FNGs however, have been put in the Emotional Headlock (EH) prior to their first post, and we often look to the Sponsor for nicknaming guidance in the COT. (Sponsors who EH people and then don't accompany them to their first workout generally get abused.)

In addition to having someone there to guide the Q in the right direction, nickname-wise, it also helps to have a Sponsor there because otherwise an FNG might be tempted to reject his

F3 Name (hoping for a better one) or even try to use a nickname he got in college or something. Bad move.

> ### Be Careful What You Wish For ...
>
> *It's an F3 rule that guys who complain too much about their initial nickname get something worse on the second go-round. Jim Cotchett was a 1/1/11 guy whose last name reminded Dredd of Davy Crockett, so he got nicknamed Davy. He complained about it so much that he got renamed "Crotch Rocket." Same with Jason Burgess, a former walk-on basketball player at the University of North Carolina, whose original name was "Cowbell." He got renamed "Assless Chaps." Or you might get renamed with a chick name, like John "Cindy" Crawford. (For some reason, a lot of the chick-named guys are also great athletes – we've never determined the reason for the correlation.)*

As we like to say, 100% of guys who post to F3 come for the First F. Fitness – more specifically, the idea of a free Workout — is the point of entry for every guy who comes in our (nonexistent) door. It is the magnet that attracts new members to F3. Done regularly, the F3 Workout will get you in shape and keep you in shape.

To be honest, at first, you will hate the Workout — both the physical exertion, which can be extreme, and the brain-spinning lingo of F3. You might even Splash Merlot. There is an F3 word for almost everything, and most of them involve an explanation that nobody will stop and give you. But that initial drinking-from-a-firehose feeling only lasts a week or two. We have found that FNGs get the hang of it pretty quickly. And then they get addicted, not so much to the First F but to the Second F.

What keeps them coming back to the Workout is Fellowship. That is the glue of F3. Why? We are not exactly sure, but we think it has something to do with the loneliness inherent in the Problem, which we will unpack later. But we've seen it work over and over again. A guys makes his first Post, Splashes Merlot, gets mocked

Solving a Problem We Didn't Know Existed   PART 1

and slapped on the back, and gets an F3 Name. As he drags his Six back to his car, the veterans say to each other, "Well, we'll never see that dude again." But they do — sometimes the very next day. And the next.

Once in shape enough to talk and understand the F3 Lingo, that guy, former-FNG that he now is, starts Second F-ing with the other PAX and getting a good snootful of the loneliness cure. After only a few weeks, he's one of the veterans standing there after the COT watching some other FNG drag his Six back to the car.

FIRST F

SECOND F

THIRD F

Often, that's when the Third F clicks in. That's the Faith piece of it. This part of F3 takes the most effort to explain, and we attempt to do so in Part Three.

The Third F does not refer to any particular religion or worldview. It simply means that one has a concern outside of oneself. Go back to our former FNG, now an F3 veteran watching some other FNG go through what he just experienced. Suddenly, a light goes on in his head. He decides he is going to (he has to) EH his brother-in-law and some guy from work so they can be FNGs and Splash Merlot just like he did. He likes this new feeling he has so much that he wants to (he has to) share it with men who don't have it. It's that simple.

This impulse to EH another man who needs F3 in his life is what we now call the Third F. It starts at the transition point where a man stops thinking primarily of himself, where his concern becomes primarily external and in service of other men. If he follows through, he will have an impact on their lives. His transition from Survivor to Servant (another process we'll talk about in Part Three) will fill him with purpose and a drive to continue having an impact. When the men he serves and impacts in turn cross the same transition point and become servants themselves, the effect is dynamic. We have seen it happen, repeatedly. It is this dynamic effect that has caused F3's membership to explode. The First F is the magnet. The Second F is the glue. The Third F is the dynamite.

True Story: An FNG Posted one morning, Splashed Merlot, and otherwise (in his mind, and only in his mind) disgraced himself. At the end of the Workout he got his F3 Name in the COT and was dragging his Six back to his car when he stumbled accidentally into the Workout Q, who was obliviously admiring his pecs in the window of his Lexus. The FNG must have felt a little goofy because he went ahead and blurted out what was on his mind. He apologized for "slowing the group down." The Q laughed and replied that he hadn't slowed anything down. "Anyway," the Q told the FNG, "Brother, you're the reason we are here in the first place. You are why we are here."

FORTY-THREE FEET OF GOOD ROAD

A S WE SAID EARLIER, a few of us started the Mothership on 1/1/11 with only the vaguest idea of what the Problem was and not much of a grasp on the solution. We just sent e-mails to the eighty or so men we thought might like to try it. Some responded, and some didn't. We had no idea how many guys would Post that first Saturday morning. We would have been happy with five. If we could get a solid core of five men, we thought we could build that up to about twenty by the end of the year. So we were surprised when thirty-four men Posted for that inaugural session of the Mothership, in the early morning on New Year's Day.

We thought that the first Saturday's success might be an anomaly or just thirty-four guys with short-lived New Year's resolutions, so we were only cautiously optimistic about the second Saturday. Until

---

F3 Lingo (cont.)

Gloom: *Generic term for the early morning hour at which F3 Workouts usually take place and the generally dark conditions in which they are conducted.*

Fart Sack: *A man who rises and Posts in the Gloom must almost always leave the warmth and comfort of his Fart Sack to do so. Also can be used as a verb, to describe the action of missing a workout to stay in the Fart Sack, as in, 'Sorry I missed you -- decided to fart sack this morning.'*

we saw thirty-something men gathering again in the Gloom. The third Saturday was the same. By the fourth Saturday, we realized we were onto something. In a month, we had far exceeded our expectations for the year. That was wonderful, but it also created a problem for us. We had expected to use that year to figure out how to run the group, but this early and unexpected success forced us to improvise quickly so we wouldn't squander the opportunities it created. This has been the pattern for us ever since, improvising to capture opportunities. It has seemed to us like we have been scrambling to build a road forty-three feet in front of the men driving on it.

Given that challenge (and the fact that we are not very creative men), we have to (ahem) "borrow" some road-building ideas from other sources. So, when a PAX asks, "Hey, have you guys ever seen *Fight Club?*" Or says "Wow, this reminds me of AA somehow." Or says, "Hey, have you guys ever read *The Starfish and the Spider?*" "Uhhhh," we respond, "Yeah, we have." All that and more. We will use any tool we find helpful.

We are not ashamed to incorporate and adapt a good idea to our needs just because we didn't come up with it. Likewise, we are not afraid to abandon something we actually did come up with ourselves if we discover that it doesn't work. This is how we have built (and keep building) the road, on the backs of the ideas of men far smarter, more creative, and more inspired than we are. This even goes for the original idea itself, which we inherited from another workout group called the Campos.

This borrow-improvise-discard method reminded Dredd of a military strategy course he took twenty years ago. The final exam had only one question on it: "Was Napoleon evolutionary or revolutionary, and why?" The obvious answer seemed to be revolutionary. This Corsican artillery captain had run headlong over every decent army in the world. He was a firestorm. Of course he was revolutionary. But the "why" part of the question was more difficult to answer, because Napoleon hadn't actually

Solving a Problem We Didn't Know Existed

PART 1

22

invented anything. He had only excelled at recognizing the good ideas of other men and putting them to work to win battles for his army. He cared more about winning than he did about innovating. Napoleon was not an agent of revolution at all; he was a master of evolution. His success was founded upon the unabashed use of other men's ideas to accomplish specific goals. He was a road builder, and he didn't care where the asphalt came from as long as it was durable enough to drive on.

Out of necessity, we have developed F3 in a similar fashion. When our road has hit an obstacle, we have not been afraid to look anywhere for a way to overcome it. If it works, we keep it. If it doesn't, we don't. F3 is a band of evolutionary pragmatists, focused on keeping forty-three feet of good road between us and the men we are serving.

CHAPTER 4

HALF THE MISSION

EVERY ROAD, NO MATTER how pragmatically constructed, needs a blueprint of some kind. F3's blueprint is in the form of its stated Mission, which is: *To plant, serve, and grow men's small workout groups, in order to reinvigorate male community leadership.* The Mission drives everything F3 does and guides its leaders in determining what F3 does not do. Without this clearly defined Mission, it would have been impossible for F3 to stay on course as it has grown. We could not keep building the road without the Mission. We wouldn't know where it is going.

Despite the importance of the Mission to F3's success, it was not yet defined when F3 was born at that New Year's Day workout. In fact, we started the Mothership with nothing more in mind than to capitalize on the success of the Campos.

The Campos is a bootcamp-style group that started in Charlotte in 2006 at a place called Freedom Park. The name Campos (Spanish for "field") derived from bilingual signs the city posted in the park that read "campos cerrado." In other words, the "fields are closed" (ironically) in Freedom Park.

Ignoring the irony of those signs (or, perhaps, embracing it), the men of the Campos turned the fields of Freedom Park into an outdoor gym that was publicly accessible and unfettered by the rules, fees, and political correctness that they saw hamstringing pay-to-play indoor gyms and the YMCA. Sure, the city could put up a sign that said the fields of Freedom Park were closed, but it couldn't stop the Campos from gathering there to work out together at 6:50 in the morning. There was nobody awake to do the stopping. The name and location were a great play on words, and the Campos was a great workout that met every Saturday morning, rain or shine (and still does). Who would want to work out in all kinds of weather at that ungodly hour? As it turned out, a lot of men did, because the Campos steadily grew to thirty men (and one woman) by November of 2010. That success led to an unexpected problem: too many members.

Later, the Mothership would encounter the same problem. There is a point in most every F3 Workout at which the number of participants detracts from Fellowship. Because the Fellowship acts as the glue of F3, protecting and promoting the Second F is critical. Erode the Fellowship and the PAX will come unstuck from the Workout. One of the many things we learned from our time in the Campos is that the size of the group is critical to its growth and prosperity. Bigger is better, but only to a point. Past that point, bigger is worse.

Sensing that the Campos had reached that point in late 2010, its leader (Gx) made the most logical decision he could at the time. He closed the Campos off to new members. Even though we were sad about Gx's decision, because we wanted to share what we had found there with other men who needed it, we understood and agreed with it. We also saw it as an opportunity. If the Campos worked so well that it had grown too large for itself, why not start another group at the same time on Saturday morning, only at a different location? With Gx's approval, that is what we did on 1/1/11, with the limited goal of accommodating the overflow of the Campos' success.

The irony of that limited goal became apparent immediately, as the Mothership had the same overflow problem, virtually from the first moment of its existence. Thirty-four PAX Posted that first day, and the number never decreased. So while the Mothership was a success on the attendance level, it was a failure on another, because it did not stop the overflow problem. It just spread it to a new location.

Even though we were pretty excited with the Mothership's initial success, we shared Gx's belief that a workout that was too large was not a good thing. In fact, we had a specific number in mind for the point at which that occurred. For us, it was eighteen PAX. Past that point, we believed that Diminishing Returns To Fellowship ("DRTF") set in. Eventually a Workout that is consistently drawing too many PAX would come to be known as a Problematic Workout, the problem being the onset of DRTF.

> **F3 Lingo (cont.)**
>
> **DRTF:** *Acronym for Diminishing Returns To Fellowship – the concept that too large a workout group can erode Fellowship among PAX.*
>
> **Problematic Workout:** *Any F3 workout that is regularly attracting a core of more than 18 PAX.*
>
> **ABD:** *Acronym for Addition By Division – the phenomenon under which Problematic Workouts that split end up creating two stronger Workouts.*
>
> **Plant-Q:** *A man who leaves an established Workout that has become Problematic, in order to Plant a new Workout.*

The number eighteen was not calculated with any scientific precision. We simply observed that even the most skilled Q was hard-pressed to fully interact with more than eighteen men. In addition, Sponsors were less able and willing to EH their FNGs into a Workout with more than eighteen men. Which made sense. No man who has been on the couch for a long time wants to Splash Merlot in front of forty men. It's like teeing off first at a member-guest golf tournament, when all the other players are standing there waiting for their turn. Most men want to get their shank out of the way in front of the smallest group possible, and it was the same for FNGs.

Moreover, the Sponsors didn't want their FNGs to get lost in the crowd. They wanted

PART 1   Solving A Problem We Didn't Know Existed

them to be intimately welcomed, the way they were on their first Post. That kind of intimacy required a small group, something (we believed) that did not exceed eighteen.

Because F3's growth has been fueled by the dynamic power of the EH, we try to help make the conditions ideal for head-locking. We encourage the Qs of Problematic Workouts to bifurcate well before any sign of DRTF. Initially, they may resist our gentle persuasion, which is not a surprise at all. It's the way all Qs (including us) have always reacted to the proposal to tinker with something that is already working very well. Why fix something that isn't broken, particularly when the Q cannot even sniff the murky DRTF he is being warned about? The Q will usually ask, "Aren't there any groups that should have stayed together, groups that were damaged when they were broken up?"

"Nope," we respond. "Not one." Every group that has broken itself up after it reached Problematic Workout status has turned into two (at least) stronger groups. That is the way it works, although we are not exactly sure why. Somehow bifurcation sharply reduces the DRTF and reenergizes the PAX of the two, now smaller, groups to double down on the EH effort. Maybe they are inspired to build back up into the Problematic Workout range all over again, but that is just a guess. We do know that this effect, what we call Addition By Division, takes place, and it usually happens pretty quickly, sometimes within the month.

Gx's solution to DRTF, to close the Campos off to new members, led us to plant the Mothership and inadvertently give ABD a shot (before we actually knew about its existence). And it worked. Since we didn't know that is what we were doing, we can't claim to have invented ABD. Nor can we claim that was our intent in planting the Mothership. Truly, we had no purpose in mind other than to accommodate the Campos' remarkable success by taking on its overflow. Within months, we were enjoying our own initial success and trying to ignore the fact that we had our own Problematic Workout on our hands.

At that point, knowing we had to bifurcate the Mothership, we began searching for a man among the PAX of the Mothership who would be willing and able to act as the leader of Mothership II. This proved to be much more difficult than we anticipated.

Furthermore, in the midst of our search for the right Plant-Q, we were distracted by a completely new problem, the one that actually forced us to define F3's Mission. It started with some of the Mothership PAX wanting to do things together that had nothing to do with working out in a parking lot in the Gloom. At first we ignored these things, thinking (and hoping) they would go away. But they didn't. We started referring to the things as "opportunities to succeed" or just Opportunities, because we didn't actually believe they were. We thought they were distractions, even when they were objectively positive for the community, like building a Habitat House together or partnering with Junior Achievement or leading an anti-bullying initiative.

At first we were bewildered. We had no organization. We had no structure. All we did was work out together in a parking lot in the Gloom. Why did these PAX think we could do anything else? When a PAX proposed an Opportunity, we would think, "Sure, we could do that. But why? What does it have to do with the Workout?" We had a hard time answering that question.

Eventually, we felt like we had to stop ignoring the Opportunities and at least pretend to address them. We started by asking the Opportunity-proposing guy what we had been asking ourselves: Why should we build a Habitat House together (or whatever it was he wanted to do)?

We found that these well-meaning Opportunity-proposing PAX couldn't articulate a why any better than we could, other than to say that we were a bunch of guys who could do things together (the Workout proved that), and that he cared about the homeless (or whomever) so much that he just assumed it would be a good idea for everybody. That was about it. Basically, that the Opportunity should be done and we could do it.

Well, sure, we agreed, it was a good idea for anybody who shared his level of concern for the homeless (or whomever) but not necessarily everybody does. A lot of guys don't care about the homeless any more (or less) than they care about starving children or any other group of people (or animals) with a specific need or problem. So, it didn't naturally follow that the other Mothership PAX would be as committed as this guy was to building a Habitat House (or whatever). Maybe most of them just wanted to work out together. We didn't really know. We thought our primary problem at the time was DRTF, and this Opportunity thing was keeping us from solving it.

Also, we were afraid that if we spent too much considering (or pretending to consider, as the case may have been) all these Opportunities, we would lose focus on the central purpose of the Mothership (which we had yet to actually define). Do that long enough and the Mothership would become like a rudderless ship steaming in circles until all the passengers jumped off because it wasn't going anywhere. Although it was early in the life of the Mothership, we thought we were onto something special, something different than what were getting out of other activities we participated in, like our churches and other social organizations. We didn't want F3 to end up drifting aimlessly until it became a ghost ship.

We could see all that clearly enough. The problem was how to articulate it effectively to the PAX we loved who kept throwing Opportunities at us. Thinking this problem through, we realized that that we were coming at it from the wrong end. We couldn't protect the Mothership from the things it did not do until we defined what the Mothership actually did do, and why it did it.

The search for F3's WHAT and WHY led back to the need for a permanent solution to DRTF. The Mothership was a Problematic Workout. It numbered in the high thirties every week and was growing. We needed a Plant-Q to do what we had done at the Campos – leave and start a new Workout. But nobody seemed likely or willing to do that. And, if the Mothership was any example to go by, it wasn't a long-term solution. The Mothership II was likely to have the same overflow problem the Campos and the Mothership had. We needed something more aggressive. We needed a way to scale out what was working at the Mothership to as many men as possible.

We considered a lot of possible solutions to DRTF before we succumbed to Occam's Razor and accepted the most obvious one. If we needed more Workouts, we were going to have to stop waiting for them to fall out of the sky and plant them ourselves. Furthermore, the planting was simply not going to work if done ad hoc and only in reaction to an existing Workout that was already coming loose at the seams with PAX. Workout planting would have to be deliberate, systematic, and in anticipation of DRTF. We needed to build it so they would come, not after they had already gotten there.

Figuring that out was good, but we still had the problem of not knowing how to plant Workouts. We looked around and could not find any examples of anyone having done this before. There were no good ideas to borrow or steal. All we had to look at for experience and example was the Mothership. So we did. We catalogued both the mistakes we had made when we started it, and the screw-ups we had committed trying to grow it. Counting ourselves lucky for not having killed the Mothership in the cradle, we nonetheless realized that we had learned quite a bit. At least we knew what not to do, and that alone had value. That was something we could pass on to Plant-Qs of new Workouts.

Our experience with the Mothership also led to the realization that once a new Workout was planted, the Plant-Q would need help growing it. We had learned a lot about what not to do in that area as well. Taken together, what we had learned from planting and growing the Mothership helped us define the WHAT component of our Mission, the thing F3 was supposed to do. At its simplest, this was to replicate the Mothership by planting and serving new Workouts to help them grow. Once we grasped that,

PART 1   Solving A Problem We Didn't Know Existed

we were able to distill our WHAT to this simple statement: **plant, serve, and grow small workout groups for men.**

Just writing that on the whiteboard gave us some immediate relief. Now we felt we could direct our efforts toward this specified WHAT without a huge debate about every Opportunity that came our way. All we had to ask was, "How does (insert Opportunity here) lead to, assist, or in any way help us in performing our WHAT of planting, serving, and growing men's small workout groups?" Generally, the answer was that it didn't. It was a good thing, this Opportunity, but it simply was not WHAT we do. It was not part of our Mission.

Once we had the WHAT, we turned to the WHY. It was not enough to define the task we were seeking to accomplish. We also needed to understand and articulate WHY we were doing it. We needed to define the purpose – the desired end-state – of all the planting, serving, and growing we intended to do. Building a road makes little sense if you know where you want it to go, but you don't know why you want to get there.

Why is that? As an example, take this scenario most of us have encountered in some form or fashion. Your boss walks into your office and tells you he needs a report to give to his boss on the team's results for the year. This is going to your boss's boss, you think to yourself, so you dig in. You call sales, production, finance, HR and assemble a masterpiece of a 10-slide PowerPoint deck. It's got metrics from here to next quarter, bullet points that target with deadly accuracy, pie charts and graphs that pull it all together.

You walk into your boss's office and hand it to him. He flips a couple of pages, drops it on his desk.

"Thanks, but all I needed was the sales totals by quarter. Can you just make me a slide with that chart?"

Your boss gave you the WHAT (the Task): a report on the team's results for the year. You didn't ask the WHY (the Purpose) and he didn't tell you. As a result, you didn't allocate the proper resources and didn't align your effort appropriately to the task. That's a day of work you're never going to get back, because you and your boss failed to match your Task and Purpose

Because you set out on your Task without knowing your Purpose, you misallocated resources, wasted time and, ultimately, failed. This, (unless blind luck intercedes) is the inevitable result when a man, or an organization, sets out do the WHAT without knowing the WHY. A complete mission must have both Task and Purpose.

That part (knowing you need a defined purpose) is simple. The hard part is doing the defining. In trying to define and articulate F3's Purpose (to fit with its Task of planting, serving, and growing men's small workout groups), we found that we had to first identify the Problem that F3 was trying to solve. Would the Problem be solved by a tricked out, 10-page PowerPoint deck or a simple chart of sales results by quarter? Again, that seemed simple at first, but it actually wasn't. It was actually very hard to do.

Why? One reason is that people and organizations (including us) are not actually very good at identifying problems. We don't get much practice at it and don't have a methodology for doing it.

"Really?" you ask yourself as you read this. Yes, we say.

"No, that's not right. I solve problems all day long. In fact, that's ALL I do." Sure, you solve problems. We all solve problems. That's what men do, particularly the kind of men who join F3. But solving problems is different from identifying problems, and most men don't do that all day, or at all. Mostly the problems are identified for us (or we assume them), and then we set out to solve them under the assumption that the identifier was correct. That's how you end up trying to align margins on PowerPoint decks when all you needed to do was run a simple report out of the sales database. Faulty problem identification leads to misallocated resources.

We would not be surprised if you are still shaking your head in disagreement. We thought we were good problem identifiers

Solving A Problem We Didn't Know Existed

PART 1

too, until we tried to do it. And it should have been easy for us, because the Problem we were trying to identify was already being solved by the Mothership. All we had to do was figure out what it was. But we couldn't, at least not at first. Eventually, we came to believe that we are not alone in our inability to identify the Problem. Our culture is simply not good at identifying problems, even when it is doing great and wonderful things.

Take one of the Opportunities as an example: Habitat For Humanity. It's a great outreach for a church or other civic organization. Your group builds a house for a homeless family. The group members get to take part in the construction, even if (especially if) they have never done anything like that before. The target family is right there with you, watching this happen and pitching in too. There is a real connection between the servers and the served.

To build a Habitat House, your organization will need about $70,000 to buy the land and materials, and lot of sweat and man hours to put it all together. This is all for one family to not be homeless anymore. Let's get this straight right now. We believe that this is an objectively good thing, and anybody who has the homeless on his heart is likely to be joyful in participating.

But, we asked when this particular Opportunity came our way, what exactly is the problem that Habitat is designed to solve? If you were trying to write Habitat's mission the way we tried to write F3's mission, and you had gotten past the Task (build a house for a homeless family), what would you say the Purpose was? WHY are you building a house for one homeless family?

To us, it seemed that for Habitat the problem had to be "homelessness," which made its Purpose "ending homelessness." Clearly and unquestionably that is a worthy WHY. And yet, if ending homelessness is the Purpose, then Habitat's Task (its WHAT) of building a house for a single homeless family didn't make much sense to us. Every city has voluminous unoccupied and distressed housing that could be refurbished more quickly and inexpensively, and for many more people, than just the one family Habitat helps.

Also, it didn't make much sense to us to have volunteers who had no idea what they were doing constructing the house. Why should real estate agents (for example), who would be good at finding likely properties to refurbish for the homeless masses, spend that valuable time and energy doing something they don't know how to do (like putting up drywall) for only one family?

Even our Opportunity guy himself admitted it probably doesn't make much sense when you look at it that way. "But," he pointed out, "those realtors love putting up drywall." It's empowering to them, even if it is inefficient. OK. If that's so, and we have no reason to doubt it, maybe the problem that Habitat actually solves is not homelessness, but that the homed need to feel more purposeful in their outreach to the homeless. So, even though he smashes his thumb with a hammer doing it, a realtor may be more fulfilled putting up drywall for the one family that he can see standing there, than he would be finding properties for 100 families that he never sees or touches.

Habitat might be a solution primarily for the homed rather than the homeless. Again, there is nothing wrong with that if the problem is properly identified in the first place. Otherwise there is likely to be a misallocation of resources and loss of impact. We wanted to get F3's Problem identified accurately, because it seemed to us that any solution designed for a misidentified problem had to be doomed to failure.

Ultimately, as difficult as it was, we were able to pin down the Problem F3 was solving. It took more than one whiteboard session. And, we found it to be far more complex than we had expected, too complex for one chapter in this book. In fact, it fills the entirety of Part Two.

Solving A Problem We Didn't Know Existed

PART 1

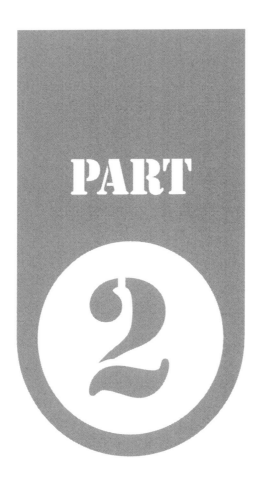

PART

2

THE PROBLEM

1

A GOOD PLACE TO STOP

STOP READING FOR JUST a second. We appreciate that you've gotten this far, but this might be a good place for you to stop and go do something else. This may not be for you. We tell you that because we don't like to waste people's time. We are busy men and assume you are busy too. This is a good point for us to take a page or two and tell you what the rest of this book is not, so you can make an informed decision whether to keep reading it.

First, this is not an exercise book. You won't find any revolutionary ideas in here or fancy workout routines. F3 is about Fitness, not exercise. We don't have much to say about getting in shape. We are far more focused on staying in shape. Getting in shape is a sprint fueled by the enthusiasm of a change for the better, but staying in shape is a marathon that is sustained by discipline and near-maximum effort virtually every day of a man's life. This is a central truth of F3's First F, and there is no way around it.

The Near-Maximum Daily Effort

As we mentioned earlier, we're suckers for any useful idea and have patched together much of F3 from bits and pieces that we've come across over the years. When we say that staying in shape requires near-daily maximum effort, we're speaking from experience. We both suffered from inconsistent ▶

> *fitness for years, characterized by plenty of "rest days," recurring small injuries, and changing plans and objectives that led to yo-yoing weight. The level of fitness that we found – and sustained – once we stumbled into the F3 model changed all that for us and was further confirmed by a book we encountered at the Campos, Younger Next Year, whose authors argue convincingly that WHAT you do for exercise matters far less than HOW OFTEN (every day) and HOW HARD you do it.*

Most exercise books (of which this is not one) offer magical shortcuts around the truth. If anyone ever comes up with one that works, we'll be early adopters. We hate the truth too. It hurts. But there is no shortcut. You have to make what we came to call in F3 "the daily down-PAINment." The good news (which is much of what the rest of this book is about) is that you don't have to do it alone. In fact, it's almost impossible to do it alone. That's the point of the Workout. Not just to do it, but to not do it alone.

The bottom line is that if you are looking for a magical exercise shortcut, put this book down. It won't help you. But if you are ready to accept reality and want to know what you can do about it, keep reading. We think F3 can help you. It helped us.

The next thing to know is that this book contains no great social insight. We love the Malcolm Gladwell thing and will be citing him later. But we are not here to reveal the underlying mystery of why men live as they do without seeming to like it. What we are is livers (men who live, not the organ) who stumbled upon a more purposeful way to do it. We will describe that way with little or no reasoning as to how we got to the sorry state we found ourselves in. We don't point any fingers. We don't care whose fault it is or was. If you are looking for that, don't read the rest of this book. You will be disappointed. There are lots of other books on the shelves that will do that for you.

This is not a book about religion. There is no theology here. Yes, the Third F is Faith, but we don't believe that's the same thing as religion. We will not be answering the great questions of man's origin in here. We are not offering a new path to enlightenment or attacking any of the old paths. We do have personal beliefs, which we may refer to obliquely from time to time, but only to give context and not as part of an effort to convince you to believe the same. That being said, we do believe that everyone believes something, but that is about where that ends. So, if you are looking for a theological treatise (or the opposite), don't bother reading another word. Put the book down now and paint your shed.

Finally, this is not a story of anyone's personal struggle and ultimate triumph. For starters, we're still struggling (although we are much happier about it now). More importantly, there is no trophy-hoisting moment in here. We are not describing a plateau of grandeur to which you can climb and perch for the rest of your life with struggles past reduced to distant memory. It's all a mountainside that you either climb up or slide down, a little bit every day. What we want is to explain how F3 may be a better way for you to keep climbing. The plateau thing? That's a myth. If you are looking for that unicorn, don't go any farther than this page.

Don't get us wrong. We want you to read every word we have written. Partly out of pride, but also because we think it might help you the way it has helped us and a lot of other men we know. We just don't want you to get to the end and ask, "What the heck is this thing? I don't care about any of this. I wanted to read about the Dalai Lama's Enlightenment Gained Through His Struggle To Complete P90X." That's not what this book is at all. Not even close.

The Problem

PART 2

SADCLOWN SYNDROME

S O WHAT IS THE Problem? We call the Problem "SadClown Syndrome." We were SadClowns. We know what it feels like. We have met a lot of SadClowns. We know what it looks like. When we set out to define F3's Purpose, WHY F3 did WHAT it did, we discovered that F3 was solving SadClown Syndrome.

For starters, it's a man thing. We are not saying women don't have problems, or even that they don't have this particular problem. We just don't know much about women's problems. Despite having many years of marriage and several daughters between us, we are happy to admit that we have only a mere inkling as to what makes women tick. We have found that we serve the women in our lives best by being good husbands and fathers. That is (in part) what F3 is about. So, we are sticking to what we know here, and that is men. Men, we believe there to be many, are suffering from SadClown Syndrome. We're pretty sure we are right about that.

How many exactly? We don't know, and, frankly, that's irrelevant to us at this point.

What convinces us (without backup data) that the Problem is widespread enough to justify a book about it? Just what we see right in front of us. We planted the Mothership on 1/1/11. It was cold. It was 0650 in the morning. Everybody was a little hungover. All we did to advertise the Mothership launch was to send out a few emails to guys we thought might Post, and thirty-four men climbed out of the Fart Sack to do it. They must have been looking for something.

One guy (that we saw) Splashed Merlot, and a lot of the others complained the entire time. Yet, the following week, most of those guys Posted again. In fact, most of those guys are still with us today, three years later. So are thousands of other guys who joined after that first day. We think we are onto something. We believe SadClown Syndrome is real, widespread, and that F3 has caught on because it offers a solution to it.

We didn't make up the "SadClown" idea. It comes from an episode of *The Sopranos*, the HBO series that depicted a suburban New Jersey Mafia family stripped of the gothic grandeur of *The Godfather*. The primary character of the show was the leader of the family, Tony Soprano. Although his livelihood was criminal, Tony had leadership dilemmas and work-family stress problems just like the average man. Just like us. He even had a psychiatrist, Dr. Melfi, whom Tony began seeing when the fainting spells that had plagued him since his childhood became too dangerous for him to ignore.

Tony's sessions with Dr. Melfi were the vehicle to reveal his underlying character and motivation. Initially, with his limited therapeutic goal of curing his fainting, Tony was guarded with Dr. Melfi. But as the series progressed, Tony began confiding in her more deeply than anyone else in his life. She became the only person in his life with whom he could be safely and completely truthful.

Like a lot of guys we know, Tony lived a compartmentalized life. He kept his work life, his family life, his love life, and his creative life in separate vaults. *The Sopranos* did a great job of illustrating this in ways with which we only could partly identify. For example, one episode has Tony visiting a prospective college with his high school daughter when he is forced to take a quick break to kill a man with a garrote. Five minutes later, he is eating finger sandwiches with his daughter. That is serious compartmentalization.

Most men are forced to balance their work and their family lives, but not to Tony's extremes. For him, there was a massive tension in the fundamental contradictions of his life which, as he began to trust her, Dr. Melfi tried to help Tony reconcile.

During the episode that gave us the "SadClown," she asked Tony if he had "any qualms about how you actually make a living?"

"Yeah," Tony responded. "I find I have to be the sad clown: laughing on the outside, crying on the inside."

Tony missed the doctor's point. He did not understand that she was asking him to reflect on a possible connection between his fainting and his gangster livelihood. He understood her to be asking him if he liked his compartmentalized life, and he answered like any discontented banker or lawyer would. No, he told her. No, I don't like it all. I only pretend to like it because I feel like I have to.

Despite his family and the career success (such as it was) that he had clawed out, Tony was not happy. He only pretended to be happy for self-preservation and for the benefit of the people who depended upon him. Internally, he was joyless. But that, his true condition, he kept from everyone except Dr. Melfi, a woman he paid by the hour to listen to him. Only to her would he admit that he was a SadClown.

Because he was smart and devious, Tony managed to stay out of prison, but to what end? His life was a prison. He was a fat, friendless middle-aged man who self-medicated with booze and womanizing. He was plagued by fainting spells that threatened a life and livelihood that he had to fight (literally) to preserve, even though he could see no purpose in it other than its very preservation. What kept us watching such a depressing show was our hope that Tony would find a way out of his SadClown prison. But he never did. He remained a SadClown until the end.

3

BOWLING BALL GRIP

Like any affliction, SadClown Syndrome has some identifiable symptoms. We group them into a single manifestation we call The Bowling Ball Grip. It consists of three holes in a man's life that render him as inert as a forgotten bowling ball in the back of the family junk closet. A bowling ball is made for impact. It is supposed to be in motion, to roll fast and knock down pins. But it cannot do that on its own. Unless somebody fills its holes and hurls it into motion, it will only sit and gather dust.

Before F3, when we were SadClowns, we were like those dusty bowling balls, but we didn't know it. That's because a man can't see the holes of his own Grip while they remain unfilled. He can only feel their effect on his life in the form of a vague but nagging lassitude and dissatisfaction. That's the gathering dust. SadClown Syndrome compels a man to hide this dissatisfaction with the things of his life that he knows should bring him joy. It leads him to hide the Grip even from himself.

What our culture calls a mid-life crisis is actually a SadClown's effort to self-prescribe a remedy for his joyless inertia. Instead of filling the holes of the Grip he cannot or will not see, the SadClown sees what he can in his life and declares his circumstances to be the cause (rather than the effect) of his malaise. As a result, the SadClown concludes that he is a man whose wife and job are making him unhappy when, in fact, he is an unhappy man with a wife and a job.

No surprise then, that having misdiagnosed the problem, the SadClown proceeds to the wrong solution. If he's bold (or reckless), that might mean divorce and a career change. If he's meek (or careful), that might mean porn and workplace malingering. In between, there are a whole range of self-medicated solutions that are equally ineffective because they do not fill the Grip. They do not solve the Problem.

We've given names to the Bowling Ball Grip's three holes: Pogo40, The Sifter, and The Reacher. We told you before that we're not psychologists or social scientists. What follows here is not based on any kind of learned study or controlled experiment, only on our observations as recovering SadClowns and beggars who want to show the others where we found our crumb.

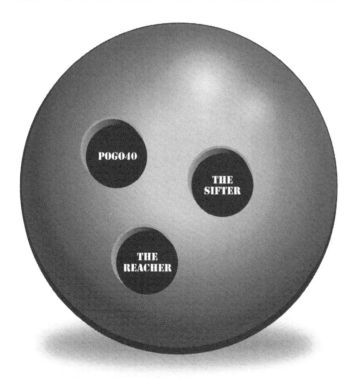

CHAPTER 4

POGO40

THE FIRST HOLE OF the Grip is Pogo40. It is about a man's physical fitness, or rather, his inconsistent physical fitness. The name derives from the forty (or so) pounds a SadClown keeps losing, only to gain back again. Over and over.

Pogo40 is not the static morbid obesity of a fat man who makes no effort to change. That's a different problem. In Pogo40 there is no stasis. The afflicted man is either climbing toward "Good Shape" (forty pounds down) or sliding back down to "Fat Pants" (forty pounds up). Although he never reaches a point of equilibrium, he also never stops trying, thanks to the anesthesia of self-delusion. The closer he gets to Good Shape the more certain he becomes that this will be the last time he has to make this nasty climb. His belief is unshaken by the fact that this is his tenth trip up the mountain in the last twenty years. He believes that this is the time he will climb right past the peak of Good Shape to that utopian Plateau that he believes must be nestled right behind it.

The Plateau is the magical place where a man can stop climbing without sliding back down, the place where his struggles are over. Nobody has to count calories or drink Ultras on the Plateau. You don't have to spend a mind-numbing hour on the elliptical trainer every day when you reach the Plateau. You can just play tennis, stay in shape. You know, fun stuff. Just because the SadClown never gets to the Plateau doesn't mean it's not up there. What happens (he thinks) is that he always gives up just a bit too soon. Probably when the Plateau is just past the next ridge. This time up to Good Shape (he thinks), he just won't quit.

Each SadClown has his own Pogo40 routine (picture Tony Soprano sweating it out in a wife-beater on his elliptical trainer in the basement). Here is a description of a routine you may recognize. Our SadClown has lost thirty-eight pounds in three months through the same draconian diet and exercise program he always uses to climb to Good Shape. He has a routine that works for him every time: 1) he limits himself to 1500 calories a day; 2) he weighs himself every Monday on the same exact scale and at the same exact time, and records his progress in his workout diary (the Moleskin); 3) he takes his Moleskin to the gym four times a week so he can also record his weightlifting routine and twenty-minute session on the elliptical trainer.

The key to the SadClown's routine is consistency. Writing it down in his Moleskin really helps. While he's climbing to Good Shape he never varies from his routine. For that duration, he's a zealot. The routine requires our SadClown to ride the same elliptical trainer every time. That's part of his consistency. It is like territory marked with personal sweat. At some point, the YMCA helpfully planted a Fern in a clay pot right next to the SadClown's elliptical trainer, probably to dress the place up a bit. Over the years, the SadClown has grown unnaturally fond of that Fern. To him, it's become more than a potted plant, it's (sadly) his "workout buddy" of sorts.

This starts as a joke between our SadClown and his wife. As he heads out the door, clutching his Moleskin and water bottle, the SadClown says, "Gotta go see the Fern." After a couple of trips up and down Pogo40, the Fern evolves from a joke to a silent companion, like Tom Hank's volleyball Wilson in *Castaway*.

A man has to have somebody (or something) to talk to when the going gets rough. For our SadClown, that's the Fern. When he starts to tucker out on the elliptical trainer, he says, "Yeah, Fern, I'm feeling it, but I'm not going to quit. Gonna see the Plateau this time." And Fern silently urges him onward. It seems crazy, but it makes sense to the SadClown on the neighboring recumbent bicycle — he's conversing with the ficus next to his machine.

Although Fern never verbally responds (it's a plant), its silent vigil gives our SadClown the kind of encouragement he wants. Fern is the perfect companion, never asking anything from the SadClown in return for its encouragement.

The only other participant in the SadClown's lonely climb is Crystal, the YMCA-certified-personal-trainer that the SadClown's wife gave him as a present one Christmas when he was deep in his Fat Pants. Once a week, Crystal makes our SadClown do lunge walks around the YMCA mini-track and bunny hops up the stairs. Unlike Fern, Crystal can talk, but you have to pay her to do it. Which our SadClown does. He doesn't mind paying her to talk. The downside is that when he stops paying her, she stops talking. The choice is up to SadClown.

While SadClown's routine is all monotonous rigor, it has its cleansing aspect.

While he's climbing, he's hungry, and the hunger makes him oddly energetic and as close to euphoric as he ever gets in his life. The closer the scale tells him he is to losing the forty, the more confident he grows that this is the time he will find the Plateau.

It is there, right at the Pogo40's upward apex, that the power of the SadClown's anesthetic self-delusion is at its most potent. There, he always experiences a fleeting weightlessness, just before gravity sucks him back into his inevitable slide down to Fat Pants. Without that anesthesia, SadClown would be able to see that there is no Plateau, that there is only a rugged and endless upward path that must be climbed every day. He would know that once he stops climbing, he will slide until he hits bottom. Up and down. Over and over. Just like a pogo stick. That's the black magic of Pogo40.

But SadClown can't see that. His downward slide to Fat Pants begins the very day he writes down "40—Mission Accomplished!!" in his Moleskin. That's when he stops weighing himself and puts

PART 2   The Problem

his Moleskin back on the shelf. These are progress-measuring tools that he doesn't need on the Plateau. There is nothing more to measure.

Believing that he's finally found the Plateau (and fatigued from the climb), SadClown happily abandons the routine. He gives up his crazy draconian diet and starts to "eat healthy," which to him means that calories don't matter as long as what he is eating is "good" for him. Even that first donut in four months is OK because, well, he deserves it after all that hard work. Plus, he's still working out four days a week and surely must be burning off whatever he is taking in. Probably more!

One problem, though. He's not working out four times a week anymore. No longer euphoric from from his monastic routine, his weight/elliptical trainer workout begins to feel like the drudgery it actually is. Vaguely realizing he's dropped back to two gym visits a week, SadClown confides to Fern, "Man, I have to find something new, my routine is too routine."

But he doesn't find anything new and Fern has no suggestions (it's a plant). Before long, SadClown stops thinking about the decline in his workout frequency and quality. He can't see that he is sliding toward Fat Pants because he's under a different anesthesia from the one that kept him climbing toward the mythical Plateau. Now he's mainlining the pure denial that is only possible in the zero-accountability world of a SadClown.

If SadClown had a workout buddy with a pulse (who didn't invoice him monthly) things might be different. That guy might be able to say or do something that would pull SadClown out of his slide before he hit Fat Pants. But he doesn't. All he has is Fern, whose *raison d'etre* is silent encouragement, not accountability. It's a plant.

Nor is Crystal any help. She's pay-to-play. If you ain't paying, she's not playing. There's always another SadClown for her to lunge-walk around the YMCA. In fact, she knows that if she's patient, our

SadClown will be back. They all come back eventually. So, there is no thing or person to intercede in SadClown's downward slide.

Finally, when he can't button his flat-front khakis, the truth of what he's dreaded and ignored burns away the anesthesia. The SadClown is fat again. He holds his breath and gets on the scale. Yup, the 40 is back. He reaches deep into the back of his closet and retrieves his Fat Pants, those pleated Dockers with the 40-inch waistline. Pulling them over his now-chunky legs, he silently thanks his wife for not throwing them out (like he told her to when he thought he was on the Plateau).

With his Fat Pants back on, SadClown is depressed for a few days (weeks or months), however long it takes his resolve to return for another climb up to Good Shape. When it does, he dusts off the Moleskin, turns to a fresh page and writes "Day One" on top. He strokes a check to Crystal and climbs back on his elliptical trainer. Fern is still there and happy to listen. It's heard it all before.

It's a plant.

THE SIFTER

T HE SECOND HOLE OF the Bowling Ball Grip is about loneliness, the thing that leaves our SadClown with Fern (which can't talk) and Crystal (who won't talk, unless you pay her) as his sole companions.

Ah, you may be thinking, I can go ahead and skip this chapter because the last thing I am is lonely. I've got people in and out of my office all day. When I'm not working, I'm surrounded by my family. I'm coaching soccer on Saturdays. I teach Sunday School at church. I'm the opposite of lonely. If anything, I need some solitude. I'm over-peopled.

Don't skip ahead just yet.

This chapter isn't about the loneliness that comes from physical isolation. That's aloneness. This is about the emotional isolation suffered by a man without deep bonds of fellowship with other men. OK, you say, I may not have that, but I don't need it. My wife is my best friend.

We hear this quite a bit and only have two problems with it: 1) it's impossible, and 2) it's a cop-out.

It's impossible because a wife can't add best-buddy-duty to everything she already has to do in the family. Even if she could (that would be a heckuva woman), is a man really going to take all of his problems to her? Really? Aren't there some things in a man's life, some pretty important things, that require another man to address, sometimes by force? That's what accountability is about. Look at it another way. Every man needs help keeping his most important relationship, his marriage, healthy. How could his wife help him do that when she's the other half of it?

Calling your wife your best friend is a true and dangerous OprahBomb – sweet and high-sounding on the surface, but grit-less underneath. It is nothing but a stylish way for a SadClown to deny the loneliness that is keeping him inert. Like all forms of denial, it is at best useless, but a man will cling to it because it keeps him from acknowledging that his loneliness is a problem for which there is a simple but embarrassing solution: to make male friends. It's embarrassing because we can't do it. Men don't know how to make friends.

More accurately, we forgot how. Clearly, we could make friends when we were boys. We watch our sons do it now. Somehow, by the time we are adults, we lose our grasp on that elemental survival skill, in the same way we forget how to gig a frog. Rather than admit that and ask for help (man, that would be even more embarrassing), we cop out and toss out the OprahBomb that our wife is our best friend. Sound familiar?

> **F3 Lingo (cont.)**
>
> *OprahBomb: Any culturally popular sentiment with no substantive value, suitable for display on a bumpersticker. OprahBombs are always bereft of any actual standard of behavior or guidance on how to get there. Tell a SadClown to "wag more, bark less" or "turn that frown upside down." "Yeah," he'll think to himself. "I'll get right on that buddy, right after I garrote you."*

"OK," you say, "maybe you've got a point. My wife isn't my best friend. That was an OprahBomb. Forget that. But I'm still not lonely. I've got buddies." Alright, let's put all your buddies in a figurative version of the sifter your mom used to separate flour

The Problem

PART 2

50

when you were a boy. Remember how she would dump the flour in the top of the thing and shake it like crazy? What she was doing was smashing the flour against the side of the sifter so that the fine particles would pass through the screen on the bottom. What was left afterwards were the big coarse particles, those too stubborn to pass through the sieve no matter how hard your mom shook it.

This is how the strength of a man's friendships are tested when the world gives his life a good hard shake. The small particle friendships go right out the bottom of his personal Sifter. Only the big stubborn ones stick around. Be honest. Look at your male relationships. How many of them are big particle?

In our own SadClown lives we had three kinds of male friends, all of them small particle. First, is the Legacy Buddy. These are the relationships a man forms anywhere between his childhood and the last day of graduate school. In other words, before the challenges and stress of a man's real job and family kick in. Since we move around a lot, a man's Legacy Buddies often end up being long-distance friends. So even a great Legacy Buddy is still a guy you met when you were both twenty and that you have only actually seen six times since you graduated college.

No matter how often you talk on the phone or e-mail your Legacy Buddy, deep fellowship with him will be unlikely because brotherly intimacy requires physical proximity. Deep fellowship is what a man needs when his Sifter begins shaking. Most men only ask for help after they have veered clean off into the ditch, when the consequences are already in motion. In other words, when it is too late.

A large particle friend, the kind of guy who does not pass through the bottom of your life when it begins shaking, will kick you back toward the center line long before you become a Humpty Dumpty (a man who can't be put back together again). But he can only do that if he is physically present when the veering starts. He has to see it and feel it, not just hear about it over the phone (usually after the fact).

SadClown Buddies

Some of what we're going to say here about SadClown lives and friendships is going to sound harsh, but please try to remember, we're not casting blame or pointing fingers here. When we tell you that your Legacy Buddies are not sticky friends, that's not your fault or their fault and doesn't mean you love them any less or they love you any less than you did back when you were hitting keggers in the dorm. It's just reality that because they aren't proximate they can't know your life in a close-up way – and they can't intervene when things are in danger of going south.

Legacy Buddy relationships are formed at a time (the last time) in a man's life when he is culturally encouraged to form male friendships simply for their own sake. School is a time of institutionally sanctioned male-only teams, clubs, and fraternities. But that ends at the moment the mortar-boards fly. For some reason, our culture embraces the idea that a boy's school life is enhanced by friendship, but rejects that concept for a man's post-school life. Then, he's supposed to go it alone, with his wife as his best friend.

For some reason, what was encouraged in boyhood is viewed with cultural suspicion in manhood. As men, we have been willing participants in construction of culture in which all-male gatherings fall into two polar-opposite categories – either pure altruism and complete debauchery. The choice is between a church men's retreat or a drunken golf weekend – and almost nothing in between. You can help people or get some junk out of your system. But then you need to get back to work. You're a grown-up now.

If you doubt this, try starting a male-only group for no partic-ular reason and see how long it takes for someone to question why your boys club excludes women. The implication is often that male-only fellowship within the extremes of altruism and debauchery is childish and somehow unfair to women. As we said earlier, we're not sociologists, so the forces that brought this about are beyond the scope of this book. We don't know how our culture reached this point or who is to blame. All we care about is the effect it's had on men, and we believe that to be bad, very bad. Left with no post-college vehicle for forming deep, transparent friendships, it should be no surprise that men rely so heavily on their Legacy Buddies. Unfortunately, their lack of proximity makes them the first guys out of the Sifter when the shaking starts.

So let's look at a set of grown-up buddies who are proximate. We call these guys the Man Dates. They are the guys you become friends with because your wife is girlfriends with their wives. This is a lowest-common-denominator friendship and we go along with it to support our wives in their friendships, but it's really not so different from a kid playdate, is it? Everyone shows up at the appointed time. Your kid shows his playdate his trampoline; you and your Man Date go into the den and check out your big-screen TV.

As with the Legacy Friend, there is nothing inherently wrong with making friends this way. It's just that the Man Date relationship is generally too limited to stay in the Sifter when it starts to shake. There are a couple of reasons for this.

First, you and your Man Date are buddies for reasons that have nothing to do with any similarities of character, hard-wiring and interests. It's a circumstantial friendship, just like kid playdates – thrown together based on age and gender similarities, with enough toys thrown in to let the moms have a few hours of Chardonnay-sipping. That works out fine for kids. They just want to play and are happy there is another kid to do it with. When they get to school, they will make their own friends. Playdates, like Man Dates, don't last because they aren't built to last. Unfortunately, unlike our kids, we don't go on to make our own friends because our school days are behind us. Man Dates is where it stops for us.

The second reason that Man Dates fly out the bottom of the Sifter is that they are too closely cross-collateralized with the corresponding wife-relationships. When your Man Date tries to tell you his marriage is failing, you just know that you are going to get his wife's side through your wife in the very near future (probably that night). If you listen too closely to the Man Date, or are crazy enough to give him some actual sincere advice, you might then find yourself having to take his side against your own wife in a shadowbox version of their dispute in your own bedroom. To avoid that, the smart play is to not ask your Man Date too many deep questions, just nod your head and cluck like the freaking chicken you are. If you were truthful, you'd say, "Sorry, Man Date, but you're on your own now." Because that's the truth. The Man Date is flying out the bottom of the Sifter at the first sign of shaking.

The Bottom Line is that the Man Date relationship is hamstrung by an inherent conflict of interest that keeps it from staying in the Sifter when the man needs it most. It's small particle. It's superficial. All it takes is a little shaking and the Man Date is gone, baby, gone.

Which brings us to the Work Buddy, truly the low-hanging-fruit of the adult male friendship world. As with the other two Sifter-buddy groups, there is nothing inherently wrong with making friends with the guys you meet at work. But like the Legacy Buddy and the Man Date, they are nowhere near big and stubborn enough to stay in your Sifter when it's quaking.

To test this premise, think about the Work Buddies from your last job. You probably ate lunch with them a lot and played some golf. You may even have had a couples dinner with them, but probably not. (Men don't go in much for the reverse-Man Date. We like to keep our spheres compartmentalized.) That's SadClown 101. Now that you are on to your current job, do you still do see those old Work Buddies, or are you having lunch and playing golf with the guys at your new gig? Probably the latter. That's because a Work Buddy is like a guy you play pick-up basketball with at the YMCA. If he's there, great, you play with him. If he isn't, you don't hold up the game. You just play with the guys who are there. That's the whole deal with the Work Buddy. His utility is that he is locationally

PART 2   The Problem

convenient. The bond you form with him is no stronger than the walls of the cubicle between your desks.

Why? Primarily because you are in implicit financial competition with your Work Buddy. Deep male fellowship requires accountability, and accountability requires transparency. To keep you from veering into the ditch, your friend has to be able to clearly see your grimy hands on the shaky steering wheel. Transparency is not the hallmark of the work-made friendship because it's not in a man's best interest for him to reveal his flaws to his competitors. So he doesn't, no matter how badly he needs help. Even though you pick your own Work Buddy, it is a relationship that's no more built to last than the Man Date.

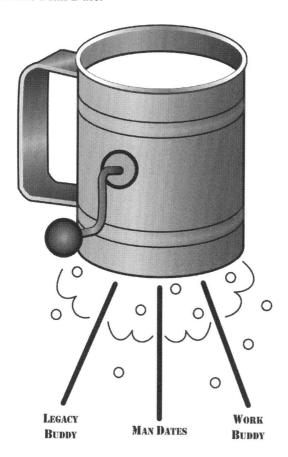

LEGACY BUDDY   **MAN DATES**   **WORK BUDDY**

Thus is The Sifter. As men, we've allowed ourselves to forget how to seek or build the kind of male-only groups in which we form deep and transparent friendships that provide us with accountability. Maybe we fool ourselves into thinking that "buddies" were something for childhood and adolescence, but that we don't need them now that we're grownups with wives and families. In our loneliness, we fall back on what's easy and available: the Legacy Buddy, the Man Date, and the Work Buddy. None of these relationships is built to last or to withstand the inevitable shaking a man's life will take from time to time.

As a result, when the sifting starts, the man is left alone when he most needs a friend. If he's lucky, he survives it more or less intact. If he's not, he becomes a Humpty Dumpty, and we know how that story ends. All the king's horses and men won't be able to help the guy then.

THE REACHER

THE FIRST HOLE, POGO40, is the up and down fitness/ fatness cycle from which the SadClown cannot seem to break free. The second hole, The Sifter, is the loneliness and lack of accountability that results from friendships too finite and frail to withstand the shaking a man's life will get from time to time. Finally, now, we have The Reacher. The Reacher is about lack of purpose.

We started writing this book before the movie *Jack Reacher* (based on a popular series of novels) came out, so we thought about changing the name of this chapter when Tom Cruise was cast as Reacher. Why? He just does not seem to physically capture the kind of lonely anti-hero man-fantasy guy who comes to mind when you read a Jack Reacher novel. But ultimately Reacher is just too good of a concept for our point about the third hole to give up on him simply because of Tom Cruise. Just try not to think about him while you are reading this.

Reacher is a 6'5", 250-pound West Point graduate who served in the Army as an officer in the Military Police corps. He is a veteran of the 1983 Beirut barracks bombing and Desert Storm eight years later. He left the Army as a major before 9/11 and became a drifter.

Reacher has no possessions. He buys a set of clothes and wears them until they are dirty. Then he throws them away and buys a new set. In his pocket are only enough cash to meet his immediate needs, an ATM card, a travel toothbrush, and an expired passport. He has no particular plan as he drifts from town to town. He lets the road or some vague notion direct his steps. Usually, he just hitchhikes and ends up where his rides are already headed.

Each Reacher novel revolves around a town (usually small and remote) into which he has inadvertently drifted. His looming presence agitates both the local good guys and the local bad guys, who are usually locked into some stalemated struggle that is about to boil over, and into which he becomes involuntarily inserted. Ultimately, the cops (assuming that they are the good guys) overcome their suspicions of his unconventional lifestyle at about the same time that the robbers (assuming that they are the bad guys) realize that he is a mortal and violent threat to their criminal enterprise.

And (of course) there is almost always a woman. She is often part of the local law enforcement apparatus. She is hard-working, lonely, somehow damaged and . . . well, you get the idea. When Reacher has set right (violently, always violently) whatever wrong was stewing in the town when he arrived, he leaves the woman behind no worse for the wear and incapable of accusing him of leading her on. After all, he's just a drifter.

In the latest Reacher novel, *Never Look Back*, the woman (a military policeman this time) asks him how much he works out (after he accedes to her request that he remove his shirt). "I don't," he answers. "It's genetic."

Yup, Reacher doesn't even have to worry about Pogo40. "No diets. No weights. No gym time," the author tells us. "If it ain't broke, don't fix it, was his attitude." Wow. What a man-fantasy that is.

There are about 18 Reacher novels, and they are all basically the same. Which is to say that they are very much like every Travis McGee novel, the entire Spenser series, the Phillip Marlowe novels, Shane, Batman, every episode of *Justified*, and . . . well, you get the idea. It's the uber-man loner-drifter with his own idiosyncratic code. The man other men love or hate (but always grudgingly admire) and women love or hate (but always yearn for). The granddaddy of the genre, America's first novel in fact, is *The Last Of The Mohicans*, and nothing much has changed since it was written. Natty Bumpo is a lot like Jack Reacher, other than 250 years between them and the fact that Natty didn't throw away his buckskins every three days.

Why is anti-hero fiction like this so popular with men? Well, like everything else that succeeds, it must be filling a need. We believe the need Reacher fills is the lack of purpose in the life of modern man. Despite our easy lives, we need something to hard to do, something to reach for. That's why we call the third hole The Reacher (it's a play on words).

A fantasy anti-hero exerts authority, but is not The Authority. He's often an ex-cop (Spenser and Reacher), a private investigator (Marlowe), or both (Spenser). If he's still a cop (Raylan Givens or Jack Bauer from *24*), he's an outlaw within, with his job hanging by a thread in every episode. Conversely, the anti-hero (like McGee and Bumpo) may have never been a cop at all (public or private) and may be living completely off the grid. Interestingly, Reacher is a combination of all forms, an ex-cop living off the grid who sometimes acts as a private investigator. He can even (like Shane) have a foot in both worlds (cop and outlaw), just as long as his general instinct is to the good. We like Reacher the most because he is the quintessential American anti-hero for all seasons. The author (of course) is an Englishman.

Even if he is nominally a cop, the anti-hero's authority never derives from the government. It comes from within. This leaves him free to exercise his authority apart from the dubious moral restraints of the government and society. This renders his (form of) justice faster and more final. It is purer and uncompromised, and since the government did not grant the anti-hero his authority, it cannot dictate to him the terms of its use. Rather, he is free to use it as he sees fit, even if that in practice amounts to little more than heroic vigilantism.

Take the television series *Justified*, for example. Raylan Givens works for the Secret Service. He is supposed to arrest bad guys. Yet he gives a murder suspect the choice of leaving town or being shot by him. The man chooses to stay, so Raylan shoots him dead. It's premeditated murder, but it's "justified" because it is consistent with Givens' idiosyncratic code. Why? The guy was a murderer.

Later, Raylan helps his ex-wife impede an investigation into her theft of $200,000 from a government evidence locker. A crime, but not a violation of Givens' personal code. Why? Because he still loves her, of course. And the money didn't really belong to anybody. And she put it back.

The beauty of the idiosyncratic code is its infinite flexibility. What's good for the goose is not necessarily good for the gander, if the gander decides it isn't. That's power. That's self-reliance. That's the exercise of manly authority, even if it really amounts to nothing but heroically-excused criminal activity.

Travis McGee lives in a houseboat. Givens lives in a transient motel. Bruce Wayne may live in a mansion, but Batman lives in a cave. Reacher? Well he lives nowhere or, in a way, everywhere. These odd living arrangements all have one thing in common: no mortgage.

McGee's description of his retirement plan was that he would make money and spend it until he was broke. And then make more money. He called that living out his retirement when he was young enough to enjoy it. Natty Bumpo didn't need money because there were plenty of deer in the forest. Reacher seems to have enough in his bank account to last indefinitely, and he steals some from bad guys when he needs it.

The anti-hero either never mentions money or seems to have plenty when he needs it. It's just not an issue.

Then there is the women thing. It is like Southern Rock music. Most of the good stuff is about the heroic ditching of a good woman. The Allman Brothers might have started it with "Ramblin' Man", but Lynyrd Skynyrd perfected it with "Free Bird".

> 'Cause I'm as free as a bird now, And this bird you can not change.

You have to love how "Free Bird" extends the garden-variety Heisman into a full-throated warning about the potential carnage that might result if a man is denied his rambling birthright. It would be like putting a bird in a cage! It's barbaric! You don't want to do that, do you, Girl? You'd not only destroy me (which I could take, sure), but you would destroy us. Isn't the memory of us better than the actual me being here? In fact, the only way we can preserve that memory is for me to turn "we" back into "me" by leaving. See, I'm doing it all for you. My freedom is the only way for me to preserve your memory of us.

"Free Bird" (and its offspring) is the anthem of the anti-hero fantasy life. Of course a man can't be tied down to a wife and a mortgage and still live purposefully. Can you imagine Travis McGee having a wife on his houseboat? Where would she put her stuff? What's Reacher going to do, let a women use his toothbrush? Shane is in love with the farmer's wife (and vice versa), and that's the primary reason he won't stay. He leaves because he loves her too much to besmirch her reputation. It's self-sacrificial to travel on, but the anti-hero is always willing to do so. His lot is a lonely but purposeful one.

To a SadClown, the anti-hero fantasy life is a complete inversion of his reality.

Whereas the anti-hero is all purpose and no restraint, the SadClown has more restraints than Gulliver strapped down on the beach, but no purpose. He's got the mortgage, taxes, speed-limits, soccer games, bosses, and mothers-in-law. The anti-hero has none of that. He won't put up with it. He just moves on (after he's done with the hero-stuff) for the benefit of all involved. It's SadClown fantasy stuff. And it's utter crap.

In reality, we are all subject to the authority of our government, our employer, and our next door neighbor who complains about our untrimmed hedges. We are not running away from our wives (her family), our family or anyone else who loves and depends upon us. We don't get to make up our own code and rules. In reality, most men want to get married to one woman (at least at a time) and stay with her through good and bad, thick and thin. We're not actually born to ramble and fly away like a bird. We are born to protect and love. We are born to stay and fight. None of us wants to live like Jack Reacher. We just want the lives we're living to mean something, to have purpose.

But that kind of purpose is hard for a man to find in world without existential threat, overrun with rampant pornography and cheap video games. Instead of reaching for real purpose, SadClowns sink into anti-hero fantasies and lose focus on the real reasons a man stays, loves, and fights for his family and community. Only by abandoning himself can he hope to re-attain this real sense of purpose. To do this, he must have faith in something he cannot see.

Of course, there is risk in that. It's safer to have the Walter Mitty dream about leaving to do huge heroic things than it is to stay and actually do huge heroic things. It's easier to fantasize about a fictional purpose than reach out for a real purpose that is right in front of you. But easier isn't better. Easier is a hole, the third hole in the Bowling Ball Grip. Together with the inconsistent fitness of Pogo40 and the loneliness of The Sifter, it keeps a man inert and gathering dust. If unfilled, it will swallow him up so deep in SadClown Syndrome that he will never find a way out.

The Problem

PART 2

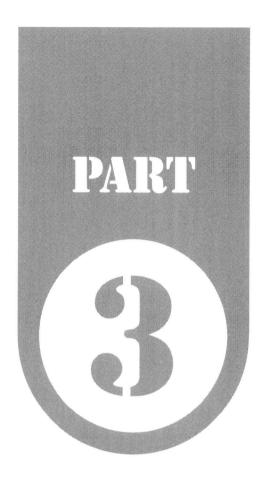

PART

3

THE SOLUTION

THE FULL MISSION

NOW THAT WE HAVE described the Problem, we can move on to the solution. Or, perhaps a solution. To be clear, we are not claiming that F3 is the only solution to SadClown Syndrome. There could well be others. Our sole contention is that the application of Three Fs in the life of a SadClown has a reinvigorating effect. It fills the three holes in the Bowling Ball Grip, picks the man up and puts him in motion. Once that occurs, we believe that it is inevitable that the man will have an impact of some kind on the world around him, whereas before, in his SadClown state, the man had none. He was inert and gathering dust.

This accelerating impact we see is different in each man. It is based on his hard-wired skill set and the concerns of his heart. He becomes missional, and the mission is one unique to him. Much as a bowling ball is made to roll down lanes and knock down pins, each man is made for something. F3 is the hand that puts the ball in motion. It knocks the dust off and helps the man find his lane so he can begin rolling again. It helps him be what he was designed to be.

Having determined the Problem and identified how F3 was solving it, we were able to finish our mission statement by defining F3's Purpose. We did this by imagining men freed from SadClown Syndrome. We envisioned men having an impact on their families, workplaces, and communities. Although that impact would vary by the man, we did not have to search long for the word that would encompass it in all forms. The word was Leadership. If SadClown Syndrome was the problem of individual man, the collective problem in the community of SadClowns was a lack of male leadership.

We believed this because, by definition, a SadClown cannot be a leader. There are many different forms of leadership, but all of them require some kind of movement and impact. Obviously, it is not possible to follow an inert SadClown because he isn't going anywhere. Nor can a SadClown himself be a follower because he is incapable of movement. His inertia keeps him rooted. Thus, a community of SadClowns is one in which there are no leaders, no followers, and no movement. At best, it might have institutionalized leadership that has learned to mimic motion so that it can appear to have impact. This is SadClown Mascot-leadership. The best mascots have the most realistic looking costumes, but the effect (or lack thereof) is the same. At the end of the day, a Mascot-leader is no more a danger to the inertia that besets his community than a man dressed up in a bear costume is a danger to a picnic basket.

When we looked around at our families (including our own), our churches, our workplaces and our city, we saw the communal inertia caused by SadClown Syndrome. In places it was partially obscured by Mascot-leadership, but it wasn't hard to see the underlying decay.

This was why, despite how much they annoyed us at first, the Opportunities that guys were bringing to us at the Mothership were so important. F3 had filled the Bowling Ball Grip in these men's lives. They were in motion now and, being Bowling Balls, they wanted nothing more than to have impact, to knock down pins. They wanted to lead and to follow.

This unleashing, we realized, is F3's end-state and Purpose: the reinvigoration of male leadership within the community. This was the WHY to the WHAT that F3 did. Now we had the other half of our Mission and could put it all together. F3's Mission became to plant, grow, and serve men's small workout groups in order to reinvigorate male community leadership. Once established, our Mission became F3's sword and shield, directing our efforts and protecting us from non-missional distractions that sap energy and resources.

The Mission provides the men who have joined F3 with a star to follow in the Gloom. Without the Mission, F3 is nothing but a gym. A crazy kind of gym, but a gym nonetheless. And we believe it to be much more than that.

THE MAGNET OF THE FIRST F

T HE FIRST F FILLS the first hole (inconsistent fitness) of the Bowling Ball Grip. When a man starts Posting regularly to a Workout, he has no choice but to get in shape. He will not need his FatPants to motivate him to get up in the morning. He will want to go. He will not need a scale or a Moleskin to keep track of his progress. He will be able to check that by looking right in front of him. If he is gaining today on the guys who were faster than him yesterday, he is making progress. Simple.

F3 Lingo (cont.)

Smoked: *The condition of being completely exhausted during the course of a workout. A really hard workout is a Smokefest, a Beatdown, or perhaps even an Epic Beatdown. If led by our friend Gnarly Goat, it might be an Epic Bleatdown.*

MumbleChatter: *The conversation that comes from those members of the PAX in good enough shape to keep up a running commentary about what is going on even during a workout.*

ShovelFlag: *A shovel with a detachable American flag and pole that is planted in the ground at the start of most every F3 workout. F3 Nation's best Shovel Flags are handmade in Raider's secret underground testing laboratory.*

BackBlast: *An after-the-fact writeup of what occurred at a workout – who attended, what they did, and the funny things that happened along the way.*

He will not have to pay Crystal to make him do lunges and bunny hops. The Q will do that. He can say sayonara to Fern. Once he Posts, he is done with the silent workout buddy. Now he will have real men to push him, who will call him out when he starts to backslide and who keep up the MumbleChatter in the back of the PAX.

Most importantly, he can say goodbye to Pogo40. His Fitness will still fluctuate a bit, but Posting at a Workout will make him part of a conspiracy to defeat the tide of aging. He will no longer be climbing the mountain alone. He will not find that it is easier, but he will find that it is a lot more fun.

○ SHOVELFLAGS AND BACKBLASTS

The components of the First F begin with the ShovelFlag. Like many things F3, the ShovelFlag is borrowed from the Campos, and it is exactly what it sounds like, a shovel with a flag on it. To make one, you need three components: a long-handled shovel, an American Flag on a short steel shaft and some duct tape. Gx planted our first one for us when we started the Mothership. Since then, we have planted it in the ground as the rallying point for every Workout we do, no matter where in the world that is. On those occasions where no actual ShovelFlag is available, the Workout Q plants a Virtual ShovelFlag.

There are now an unknown number of ShovelFlags in existence. Every Workout has its own. And, in true F3 fashion, there have been many functional and stylistic improvements to the original form that Campos regulars Gx and El Esbelto devised. There are some true ShovelFlag craftsmen among the PAX and (because we are men) some stiff competition. Some of these things are works of art. And some aren't. Some ShovelFlags still use the original duct tape design, list a little bit when planted, and are a bit muddy and tattered. But they still stand.

We like to think that the variety of ShovelFlags throughout F3 reflects the variety of the PAX. Some guys are new and beautiful, and some of us are listing, dirty, and tattered. But still standing. We never let a ShovelFlag or a man hit the ground.

When a man drags himself out of his Fart Sack and drives to the parking lot or soccer field where the Workout is held, he knows the ShovelFlag will be there and that the Q and the early PAX will be rallying around it, talking smack and waiting for the Workout to start. He knows that they will welcome him into the Gloom even if he is from a different city and this is his first Post to that Workout. If he has an FNG with him, he knows the PAX gathered around the ShovelFlag will break the new-guy ice with an emotional sledgehammer. All a man needs to do is look for the ShovelFlag and the rest will happen.

F3 Lingo (cont.)

LIFO: *Acronym stands for "Last In, First Out"; used interchangeably for a member of the PAX who arrives late for a workout or leaves early (doing both would be a DoubleLIFO).*

SoftCommit: *A pledge to maybe show up for a workout.*

HardCommit: *A pledge to definitely show up for a workout.*

UA: *Short for Unexcused Absence, used when a member of the PAX no-shows at a workout.*

Q-UA: *When the man scheduled to Q a workout no-shows.*

FNG-UA: *When an FNG Posts but his Sponsor does not (also known as Posting Naked).*

TruthNugget: *A story that has at its core a small nugget of truth, but large amounts of exaggeration and extrapolation applied as breading to make the story even better.*

VQ: *Stands for Virgin Q, a man who is leading a workout for the first time.*

Weinke: *A workout script, often carried in a waterproof baggie and used by a newbie Q to give him a plan he can refer during his Workout. Named for former Carolina Panthers backup QB Chris Weinke.*

There is no stretching in an F3 Workout. You can stretch at home, or you can get to the ShovelFlag early and stretch while the pre-Workout smack talking takes place. Bottom Line: when the clock strikes go, the Q moves out, even if there are still cars coming into the lot. We call those late guys LIFOs, as in Last In, First Out (we also call guys who leave the Workout before the COT LIFOs; yup, that's confusing). We do this (start on time) because we are men and leaders, and, for us, time is important. We don't waste each other's time. If bad planning or last night's burrito has made you a LIFO, you are going to have to listen for the yelling to find the PAX. Next time, you will get up earlier or tap the brakes on the salsa.

Each workout gets a BackBlast that is posted to the F3 website as soon as possible after the Workout. The BackBlast has three required components:

- A list of the PAX who posted,
- the Thang, a section that describes what the workout was comprised of, and
- the NakedMan Moleskin, which is where the Q records notable observations from the Workout (e.g., the UAs or a MerlotSplash), adding heavily breaded TruthNuggets wherever possible.

The BackBlast has many purposes. One is to share exercises and routines with other Workout Qs. Any Virgin Q can read the BackBlast from another Workout and get a good routine to use. He can then write it down and put it in a baggie (so the ink doesn't run in the Gloom) to consult during his workout. We call that a Weinke because a VQ once taped his script to his own wrist, like the onetime Carolina Panthers backup QB Chris Weinke—a man so forgetful that he had Quarterback Sneak written on his own arm (that's probably a TruthNugget).

Another purpose of the BackBlast is to provide a way for men who are on the DL or DR to stay connected. A man who has stopped Posting for some reason will often be called out by name in the BackBlast, as in "where the heck is McNugget?" Many a man has Posted after some absence merely on the CallOut alone. That guys gets a Kotter when he returns – there is no shame in a Kotter and no Cobains are necessary. It happens to us all. It's just good to see a Brother return. Unlike Fern, we can talk and we do have cell phones. This is one of the great things about F3. You cannot slink away in the dark without anybody saying anything. We don't let that happen, because we don't want it to happen to us.

This simple thing, the accountability among the PAX that comes from the implicit delegation of the right and obligation to grab a guy who is on an extended UA and drag him back for a Kotter, is a big part of what solves the Pogo40 problem. You just can't slide down to Fat Pants when you've got 25 men calling and emailing you after you miss a few Workouts. There are other reasons why F3 kills Pogo40 (that we will go into), but this is the main one.

Another thing that motivates many men to drag themselves from the FartSack is a sense of obligation to an FNG or some other guy whom you know is struggling.

"Man," you think, "I don't feel like Posting today, but what effect will my UA have on Blue? He's my boy, but the dude is even more messed up than I am. I gotta get out there."

Funny thing is, Blue is thinking the same thing about you.

See how that works? Each man Posts for the other man, thinking he needs help because he's more jacked up. There's a crazy, beautiful symmetry there. Of course, you can still ride Pogo40 in F3. It's just really hard, unlike when you were a SadClown. In the solo gig, Pogo40 is easy and inevitable. Fern doesn't care (it's a plant) and you are a client to Crystal, not a Brother. She won't give you a second thought if you Fart Sack, as long as you stroke that check and pay her invoice.

One final purpose of the BackBlast is to share information. We share news (good and bad) in the BackBlasts so a man who didn't Post (for whatever reason) knows what is going on in the community of his Workout. We all get a million e-mails a day, so many that you just stop reading them. The NakedMan Moleskin is one place you know you can find out the quick skinny. It's a virtual kiosk that just might have your name on it.

○ TIME, PLACE, AND MANNER

Subject to the minor restraints in the Core Principles, a Q is free to structure his Workout as he sees fit. Workouts do not have to take place in the Gloom of the early morning. There is at least one out there that starts in the evening. Nor must the location be a public park, school, or anywhere else. The only requirement is that it be publicly accessible. There is at least one Workout that starts at an intersection of two city streets, under a statue of a naked lady (that's not a TruthNugget).

What drives a Q's determination of Workout time and place are the preferences and needs of the PAX he is serving. Since most of us live near parks and schools, those make good locations. Since most of us have jobs and families, the Gloom is the one and only time of our day that we know we won't be needed elsewhere. As a result, most of the Workouts are in neighborhood parks and schools during the Gloom. A Q is still free to plant a ShovelFlag in a remote forest at 10:00 a.m., but it's probably only going to be him and the squirrels at the COT. The PAX just can't get there, and getting there is the point.

The Campos started with a Saturday workout from 7:00 a.m. to 8:00 a.m. The Mothership adopted that time slot as well, as have most of the Saturday Workouts that have been planted since then. Neither the hour-long duration nor that particular time are mandatory. Likewise, the first few weekday Workouts sprang up at 5:30 a.m., and last for forty-five minutes. That became the model for the weekday Workouts that followed, but it has never been mandatory. It is simply the time slot and duration that best serves the weekday needs of most of the PAX.

The Q's imagination is the sole restriction on the manner in which a Workout is conducted. The Campos and Mothership started as bootcamps, but to those of us who have been in the military that is a misnomer. There is not much variety to the physical training program at basic training because drill sergeants are kept on a pretty short leash. A Q, on the other hand, can do whatever he wants. So, we have running-only Workouts of different lengths and speeds. We have cycling Workouts. We have kettlebell Workouts. We have Core Workouts where there is no running at all. For a while, we had a swimming Workout, but that seemed to fizzle out because you can't talk and swim at the same time, and MumbleChatter is a big part of what makes F3 fun.

There is even a yoga Workout. Although we mock (we're men), we don't judge. If the PAX will Post, than it must be serving them. That's the sole criteria of a successful Workout. The point is to get the PAX to Post.

Although the word "bootcamp" is a bit off, that is the name we adopted for the base model, or typical, F3 Workout. Mainly because we haven't been able to come up with anything better. Which is strange, because we are better at naming things than we are at inventing things. Which is strange, because we are better at naming things than we are at inventing things. Here, that is reversed, because it is the thing that is uniquely F3.

The basic structure of an F3 bootcamp is something we call Pearls On A String, or POAS – a series of shortish running segments interspersed with Circles of Pain, led by the Q.

F3 Lingo – The Workout

Pearls on a String (POAS): *Term for the structure of a typical, base model F3 workout – running segments (the string) interspersed with Circle of Pain set-pieces (the pearls).*

Circle of Pain (COP): *Basic exercise formation during an F3 workout – the Q in the center of a circle of the PAX, calling exercises and cadence.*

TenCount: *A mini-break within the workout, when the Q asks a member of the PAX to count backwards from ten while everyone gets a breather.*

Pusherama: *A COP built around a series of pushup variations.*

Six Minutes of Mary: *A base-level ab-and-core sequence. Reference is to the "6-Minute Abs" joke from the movie* There's Something About Mary.

At the end of each segment of String, the Q takes up the center of the COP and calls out a series of exercises in an order and manner of his determination. It can be a series of pushups (a Pusherama) or a set of ab and core exercises (Six Minutes of Mary). Or he can make it up as he goes along (Randerama).

The Q can use a Weinke in his COP or he can fly without wires. It's his call. Likewise, the number of repetitions of each exercise is up to him, as is the amount of rest (if any) in between each exercise. Generally in a routine, there will be at least a few TenCounts, where the Q will call out one of the PAX to count backwards from ten (or any number he chooses) to give the PAX a rest. The pace of the TenCount is up to the man called upon.

The pace of the overall Workout is up to the Q, but it must be something he is fit enough to do himself and lead

PART 3   The Solution

(a tough combination). An F3 Q does not have to be the biggest stud in his own Workout (but he should be close). However, he must be able to do everything his own Workout requires. He has to lead the way. If he doesn't, he is likely hear several calls from the PAX of "if you can't Q it, don't do it."

No PAX Left Behind

A great F3 Workout is not one that has a few SugarRays running away from a long straggle of Clydesdales. Nor is it so brutal a BeatDown that half the PAX are laying on the ground or SplashingMerlot. That proves nothing. A great Workout is one where everybody gets smoked and no man is left behind. To do that, a good Q will go Corner To Corner (C2C) with his POAS. In a C2C, the Q runs the String as hard as he can with the SugarRays to a predetermined corner (or identifiable spot of some kind) where he intends to form his COP. While the Clydesdales and FNGs are catching up, the PAX at the corner hold the plank position or do some kind of exercise until the Six arrives. At that point, the Q forms the COP and hits his Pearl with all the PAX. When the Pearl is done, the Q dissolves the COP and launches on another String to the next corner in the C2C. Lather, rinse, and repeat.

C2C seems too simple and obvious to work, but it does. By the time the Q works his way through his POAS back to the ShovelFlag, the SugarRays and the Clydesdales will be equally smoked, even though they have done the Workout at different rates and exertion levels. The workout is not dumbed down or slowed down, but no man is left behind. This is a key F3 ethic. We do not leave a man behind. Less experienced Qs will sometimes (in their exuberance) lose sight of that, but there should always be a call from a vet in the PAX to "watch the Six." In other words, don't forget the men working to catch up. Don't leave anyone behind. We do not do that.

Every Workout should get progressively and incrementally more difficult over time as the general fitness level of its PAX increases. An effective Q uses C2C to keep everyone progressing together. It works, and that is the only criteria we have in F3 for doing anything. If it works, do it. If it works really well, pass it on.

The number of Strings and Pearls, and their length and composition, varies among Workouts and Qs. There is no set standard. The primary challenge for the Q is to accommodate the range of fitness levels among the PAX who have Posted. For a Workout to be successful, the Q has to challenge both the SugarRays (light, fast guys) and the Clydesdales (big, slow guys), without driving off the FNGs and MerlotSplashers.

That's a lot of information, and you don't have to remember any of it to participate in F3. For that, all you have to do is Post to the ShovelFlag of your choice and follow the Q. Do that on more days than not, and Pogo40 is a thing of the past. It will never happen again. On the other hand, if you want to Q a Workout, the foregoing explanation might be helpful. We hope so.

○ THE STARFISH

Part of the Napoleonic road-building evolution of F3 has been devising its structure as it has grown.

Four months after F3 began, we decided to split the Mothership. As you might recall from earlier, this was a big moment for us and we thought a lot about it and planned very carefully, right down to picking the exact man we wanted to act as the Plant-Q for the Mothership II. He had been with us since 1/1/11 and rarely missed a Post. He was enthusiastic and smart. The other PAX liked and respected him. One AM we took him aside to give him the big news that he was to be the plant-Q of Mothership II and stood back so he could kiss our feet and tell us what a great opportunity this was. But that's not quite the way it went down.

Instead, while we were explaining the whole Diminishing Returns to Fellowship thing to our Plant-Q, he was nodding away like it made perfect sense and he knew exactly where we were going, right up to the moment that we told him he was the man to see it through. Then, the nodding stopped and the head shaking started. It wasn't long before he said, "You guys are nuts, I'm not doing that."

OK, not the reaction we expected. "Why not?" we asked.

"Weeeeeeeeellllllll . . . we got a great thing going here . . . don't fix something that isn't broken . . . maybe someday we could do that, but not now . . . I'm not the right guy for this . . . I'm not ready . . . how are we going to split the PAX up . . . what if nobody comes to the new Workout . . . Where are we going to do this . . . where does the white go when the snow melts . . . WhatIf, WhatIf, WhatIf . . . .?"

OK, so there was a little anxiety there we hadn't expected. Now, less than three years later, this reaction from our Plant-Q seems very quaint. This same guy has not only started and Q'd a lot of Workouts, he's convinced other men to do the same thing. Our reluctant Plant-Q has turned into a Q-machine. What happened? What changed? To explain it, we have to go back in time a little farther, to the point where we decided to plant the Mothership. At the time, we were going regularly to the Campos, where Gx was the indisputable leader. When he decided to close it off to new members, it took us a while to work up the guts to try to plant the Mothership. In truth, we had all the same questions and objections that our reluctant Plant-Q had for us. In retrospect, we realized that we saw Gx as the leader (because he was) and could not visualize ourselves in that role. And, after the Mothership got rolling, that is apparently the way our reluctant Plant-Q saw us. We were the leaders, not him. He could not see himself in that role because we were dominating the leadership of the Mothership.

That gave us a dilemma to solve. We knew that we were not going to be able to plant new Workouts without Qs willing to do it, and that we were not going to have willing Qs unless we changed the way they saw themselves within the structure of the organization. They had to see themselves as leaders before they would be willing to lead. Therefore, it was clear that the strong centralized leadership model that we inherited from the Campos inhibited growth. Yet, we were not sure what the Mothership (or any Workout) would look like without centralized leadership. If not that, then what? At the time, we were reading a book called *The Starfish and the Spider*. It was about the growth and structure of leaderless organizations. A Spider organization was the typical feudal model of pyramidical top-down leadership. On top was the king and on the bottom were the serfs. It was called a Spider because (like any arachnid) it would die if you cut off its head. A Spider had most of the power and authority centered in one leader, the head. That was a pretty good description of the Campos, and apparently the Mothership, if our reluctant Plant-Q was any barometer.

In contrast, a Starfish organization had no head or powerful centralized leadership at the top of a pyramid. It was flat, comprised primarily of appendages that were connected to a small center that did little more than hold them together. Each appendage was sufficiently self-supporting that it could be lopped off without dying. In fact, if an appendage were cut off, it would grow into a Starfish of its own, and the old Starfish would grow a new appendage to replace the missing one.

The key to the Starfish structure was for the leaders in the center to stay small and push the power, resources, and authority out to the leaders in the appendages. The book gave a diverse range of examples of Starfish organizations, everything from Alcoholics Anonymous to Al Qaeda, all of them successful both in growing and overcoming challenges in a way that a Spider simply could not.

The Campos, by choice, was a Spider. There is nothing wrong with that because the Campos was not interested in growing. That structure works very well for the Campos. But F3 is different. Growth is a major part of the Mission. If we were going to succeed in planting, serving, and growing the Mothership II (and every Workout that came after it) we needed each group to be a self-sustaining Starfish appendage. Logically, that meant that the Q of each new Workout had to be a self-sustaining leader, with all the authority and resources he needed for his group to flourish. Each Workout Q had to be big, and the center of the Starfish (what we came to call F3Nation) had to be small. We needed to create a culture and a system for transforming PAX into Qs. Since it didn't exist, we had no choice but to build it.

The Solution

PART 3

◯ **12**

Building a Q-System was not on our whiteboard when we planted the Mothership. Since we thought it would take at least a year to build up the core of the group, we intended to lead it ourselves during that time. We had no expectation of encountering DRTF within that year, so we had no expansion plan. We didn't think we would need Qs. Clearly, we miscalculated, badly. In quick succession, the success of the Mothership, the need for the Mothership II, the reluctance of our designated Plant-Q, and the determination to create a Starfish all led us to the necessity of building a Q-System. We had to create it on the fly to stay forty-three feet ahead of the fast growing PAX of F3.

We are often asked, why the letter "Q"? We borrowed that from the Campos, which was also known as the "Qrusade" (because the last name of one of the original members started with a Q, and they saw it as a crusade of sorts). Put that together, and a Campos member was also called a "Qrusader." At first, we personally ran each session of the Mothership, because everyone else was (by definition) an FNG. After about two months, some leaders began to emerge from the group, so we had them begin leading Mothership sessions. We called each man who led a session the "QIC" for that Workout. QIC (at the time) stood for Qrusader In Charge. The "In Charge" part of QIC we borrowed from the Army. There, an officer responsible for the outcome of a given mission or event was designated as the "OIC," or Officer In Charge. This was done so that there was no doubt about who had the authority over the mission and the responsibility for its outcome. We wanted the QIC to have that same feeling of responsibility and authority. Thus, the QIC was responsible for the outcome of the Workout, with the authority he needed to see it through. By the time we began to develop the Q-System, QIC had been shorthanded to "Q." So, we went with that.

The original Qs we chose to lead sessions of the Mothership had a very limited sense of their authority and responsibility, in that it did not extend past the individual sessions they were leading. That was too narrow for the Plant-Q of Mothership II. He was going to have to take care of more than his own Weinke. With few exceptions, every issue and problem at the Mothership II would be his responsibility. The buck would stop with him, without our input (mostly). To do that, he had to be big and we had to be small. That was the essence of the Q-System.

We could see that individual initiative (I2) was our Q-System's critical element. For a newly planted Workout to succeed, its Plant-Q (and the subsequent Qs he developed) would have to take whatever individual initiative was needed to grow his group into the Problematic Workout range. The question for us was how to introduce I2 into the Q-System such that Qs would put it into practice. To answer that question, we looked first to ourselves.

We had very little I2 when we planted the Mothership, just enough (and we mean just) to get it done. We did not see ourselves as independent leaders at all. If we could have done it over, as (in a sense) we were now doing with the Mothership II, what actions would we have taken to instill I2 in ourselves? Paring it down to the essentials, we stopped only when we got to the three leadership actions we believed to be necessary and indispensable to the instillation and growth of I2.

First, a leader must teach what he knows. If you want your Plant-Q to be able to do what you do without you there, you are going to have to teach him how to do it. This seems very obvious to us now that we have written it down, but we had completely overlooked it, both when we started the Mothership and when we started trying to plant the Mothership II. Of course our plant-Q was reluctant to try to do what we had done. We hadn't taught him what we had learned in doing it ourselves.

Second, a leader must make clear the mission. It is not enough for the plant-Q to be able to do the things you can do. That alone will not instill I2. To take initiative in your absence, the man must know precisely what he is supposed to accomplish. He needs to know where the ship is going if he is going to take the tiller when you leave the bridge.

That is partly why we wrote the Mission, to be a guidepost. We determined that our Qs had to know and understand the Mission if they were going to act in its furtherance on their own initiative.

Third, a leader has to reward I2 wherever and whenever he sees it, and take responsibility for any adverse outcomes that may result. Leaders always get more of what they reward and less of what they punish. No one else is going to jump out of the boat if you let the first guy drown because he can't walk very well on the water. You have to reward the effort and pull him back into the boat. This takes a lot of leadership discipline. Picture your high-school basketball coach screaming "no, no, no" as you jack up a 25-footer, and then "yes, yes, yes" if it happens to go in. That's the opposite of what we are talking about here. The shot is either good I2 when it is taken or it isn't, regardless of whether it goes in. To instill I2, a leader has to shout "yes" first if it is warranted, and deal with the missed shot afterwards without yelling "no." Otherwise, the man will only learn not to shoot unless he has your specific direction to do so. He won't take any risks. That kind of leadership environment does not instill I2, it kills it.

I2 Builders

- *Teach a prospective leader how to do what he needs to do to lead.*

- *Give him a mission, so he can know where he is meant to go even when you aren't around to tell him.*

- *Reward and praise the kind of initiative you want, regardless of the outcome.*

These I2 Builders were missing when we abruptly told our plant-Q that he had been chosen to plant the Mothership II. In retrospect, it seems like incredibly bad leadership on our part, but that is what sometimes happens when you are building the road forty-three feet in front of the men driving on it. Truthfully (incredibly), we had just expected our man to thank us for the opportunity and run out to Home Depot to buy the fixings for his own ShovelFlag. We had not provided him with any straw, and yet we expected him to make bricks. We learned that it doesn't work that way. How could it?

Having figured that out, we put the Mothership II on hold so that we could arm our Plant-Q with the I2-Builders he needed. And here is something good that resulted. Although we did our usual crappy job, it still worked. Crappy, because we had no idea how to do what we barely knew we needed to do. Yes, we taught him what we knew about planting and running a Workout (which wasn't much), and we made the mission clear to him (even though we had yet to really figure it out completely), and we rewarded even the smallest sign of I2 he exhibited (actually, we probably overdid that part a bit).

Despite the lack of guidance, it worked. Our man did plant the Mothership II. Interestingly, by the time he was ready to go, the Mothership had grown so much so that we had to do a double split into the Mothership II and III (called Latta and Mustang, but we don't want to make this any more confusing than it already is). That gave us three Saturday Workouts a mere eight months after the Mothership started, each with its own autonomous Plant-Q team and attendance ranging from 15 to 30 at each location.

Four months later (1/1/12), we launched another new Saturday Workout that itself turned into two workouts by the end of February. That is about the time that F3 began to creep out of the Charlotte Metro area. With just a little I2-Building, the Starfish had begun to spread its appendages.

○ MEAN MEAN STRIDE

As we discussed earlier, F3's Mission has both a Task and a Purpose. We plant, serve, and grow men's small workout groups for a reason beyond just to do it because it's fun. F3's desired end-state, what it hopes to achieve from all the planting, serving and growing, is

The Solution

PART 3

the reinvigoration of male community leadership. That is why the Starfish and the I2-Builder concepts are so important. For a man to be a reinvigorated leader in his family, job, church, neighborhood and city (collectively and together, his "Community"), he has to be bold and self-sustaining. To the degree he succeeds in this, he will become a man to whom others look and seek to follow. He will have impact. That's what F3 leadership is about, impact in a man's Community. There is nothing new in this idea. The cave-dwellers needed leaders, men to whom the others looked and sought to follow. Although we are not social scientists (so we don't know how it happened) it is our belief that SadClown Syndrome stripped the Community of male leadership. The men are there, but the leadership isn't. Instead of having the kind of impact a man is designed to have, we are like dusty bowling balls sitting in a mini-storage unit while the real action takes place elsewhere.

Thus, we believe, the reinvigorating effect F3 has on a man works best when it transforms him into a "modern-day warrior" like the one Rush described in their 1981 song "Tom Sawyer."

By invoking the character of Tom Sawyer, about whom Mark Twain had written a hundred years earlier, the song harkens to a very different time in America, a time when maleness was celebrated.

Tom was the quintessential boy-leader of that era. He was the kind of kid at age twelve you could see was going to have huge impact on his Community when he was a man. The book opens with Tom being punished by his Aunt Polly for damaging his clothes in a fight at school. Twain presumes that fighting is just something that boys do because, of course, it is. It's part our exuberant and hard-wired male nature. There is no mention of which participant in the fight might have been the aggressor and which the victim, so no anti-bullying classes are prescribed by Polly. Instead, she seems wholly concerned with the effect Tom's fighting has had on his wardrobe.

The punishment she devises is draconian by today's standards; she makes him whitewash a fence on a Saturday, when "all the summer world was bright and fresh, and brimming with life." This was no dwarf-sized mini-fence designed to keep labradoodles from escaping their postage-stamp front yard. This thing was thirty yards long and nine feet high, and Tom was equipped with nothing but a "bucket of whitewash and a long-handled brush." It was an all-day punishment in the hot sun and it perfectly fit the crime. In Tom's era boys could fight on Saturday but not in school. If you fought in school, you lost your Saturday. Thus, it's not Tom's warrior nature Polly is trying to curb, but his immaturity. There's a time and place for fighting, and a man needs to know the difference. What better way for a boy like Tom to learn that than to spend his Saturday painting a fence?

At least that was Polly's plan, and it was a good one. But Twain's Tom is one of those guys we have known and admired all of our lives. He is irrepressible. He never quits. Like Cool Hand Luke, you can lock up his body, but not his spirit. Tom has a warrior spirit. So, after a "dark and hopeless moment an inspiration burst upon him! Nothing less than a great, magnificent inspiration." He picks up his brush and begins whitewashing that fence like it is the only thing on earth he wants to do on that summer day. When his buddy Ben shows up ("the very boy whose ridicule he had been dreading"), Tom ignores him and keeps painting. After watching Tom paint for a while, Ben begins to mock him for having to work rather than go swimming, like Ben is getting ready to do. Tom looks at Ben and asks him, "What do you call work?" This might be work, Tom tells Ben, and it might not. Either way, "It suits Tom Sawyer." A boy doesn't get a chance to whitewash a fence every day, does he?

The hook is set, and it doesn't take long for Ben to ask Tom to let him do a little whitewashing too. But Tom, clever boy, turns him down. No, Brother, he tells him. Maybe if it was the back fence I'd let you have a turn. But seeing that it is the front fence, well, Brother, I've got to take care of this myself because he "reckons there ain't one boy in a thousand, maybe two thousand, that can do it the way it's got to be done."

Now Ben is in the net. But only after sufficient begging and bribery does Tom let him have a go at the fence. Then, "with reluctance in his face, but alacrity in his heart" he turns the brush over to Ben and plans "the slaughter of more innocents," of which there are plenty. Tom never touches the brush again that day and is paid handsomely by each boy in turn who does. Once they see Ben working on the fence, they can't help themselves. Tom may be the leader, but Ben is the first follower, and that is powerful stuff. The fence ends up with three coats of whitewash before he runs out of the stuff, otherwise he would have "bankrupted every boy in the village."

Tom Sawyer, Twain tells us, had "discovered a great law of human action, without knowing it – namely, that in order to make a man or a boy covet a thing, it is only necessary to make the thing difficult to attain." That is the difference between work and play for a man.

For us, the Great Law that Tom discovered translates into a premise of F3: Make It Hard and They Will Come. If it's hard, it's play. If it's easy, it's work. That's why we never ease back on a Workout. Hard Workouts that get progressively and incrementally harder grow into Problematic Workout status. This is both counter-intuitive and counter-cultural. Yet, we believe it to be exactly true. We have seen it. Unfortunately, in our modern life of ease there is very little that is hard. Most of us face no existential threat more dangerous than choking on a chicken wing. As a result, any man who wants to be a modern-day warrior has to deliberately search for the hard things in life (if he wants to play) or everything he does will be easy (and thus work). If he doesn't do that, if he doesn't search, then it's all work and no play, and that makes Jack a dull, soft and inert man. It makes him a SadClown.

So how does a modern-day warrior go about that? How does he find the hard things and avoid sinking into SadClown Syndrome? For starters (like Tom Sawyer) he refuses to let that initial moment of despair overcome him. He doesn't accept the imprisonment of his warrior-spirit without a fight. Then, he looks for something difficult to attain, a mission, something hard, something that demands the skill and passion of a man who as a boy had a hero's heart and has never lost it. He knows he is on the right track when whatever he is doing results in dire warnings from the well-meaning who are alarmed for his safety. He knows he's got something when they stop warning him and just try to stop him altogether.

We know what a SadClown looks like (unfortunately), but what would a modern-day warrior look like as he goes about the business of finding hard things? We think he would look the way any man would look while stalking through his community with Mean Mean Stride, yelling at the top of his lungs and refusing to wear a safety helmet while he does it.

He would look like Today's Tom Sawyer, a guy able to persuade other men to pay him for the privilege of whitewashing his fence. Not because it's easy and any man could do it, but because it's so hard that maybe only one man in a thousand, maybe two thousand, can get it done. That's what Today's Tom Sawyer looks like.

He's the kind of man who says, screw the easy way. To hell with what the culture says. Don't slow down, speed up. Follow me! I'm taking the hard path. You take the easy way, in fact you probably should. The rest of you, the one-in-two-thousand-guys, you come with me. We've got hard play to get after. Aye!!! Aye!!! Aye!!!

○ THE MUSEUM OF FAILURE

Instilling I2 in a man using the I2-Builders is both art and science. The Qs who do it best exhibit the Mean Mean Stride of a modern-day warrior. They implicitly understand Tom Sawyer's Great Law and inspire men by challenging them with the hard things they have discovered for themselves. These are the Qs who sharpen other men like iron sharpens iron. They are the backbone of the Q-System. Sharpening a man is a gradual process. If the stone is too quick or hard, it can snap the blade. Patience is required, because it can take a long time for a Q to teach a man what he knows. How long depends in part upon the junior man's starting point. The farther back it is, the longer the process takes. Some of us started a long way back, and have had a long, long road.

This was certainly true for Dredd, who was in the Army before he became a SadClown. He was twenty-one years old when he joined. The first place they sent him was Fort Benning. That's the Army's home of the Infantry. When Dredd got there he knew very little about leadership or how the Army worked. He had been in ROTC but had not really taken it to heart. Luckily, for him and the soldiers he was to eventually lead, he was at Fort Benning for a full year of training before his first assignment. The Army was serious about making sure he knew what he was doing before he tried to do it. Otherwise, he could have gotten some young men killed.

The first thing they taught Dredd at Fort Benning was how to lead physical training (PT). There was a system to it. You don't just stand in front of your platoon and tell them to do pushups until they get tired. First, he learned to put the men into the proper formation for PT, the PT Formation. There were several sub-steps to this, which all had to be done in a particular order and initiated with the correct command. These commands were complex and arcane. They were hard to memorize. But he had to do it. You couldn't just write them on a Weinke or a cheat sheet. It was usually too dark to see during PT.

Once the men were in PT Formation, Dredd was taught to begin leading them in the exercises. There were several sub-steps and commands involved in this as well. Again, you couldn't write them down, you had to know them. During the conduct of each exercise, the number of repetitions was counted by the men, while the leader kept the proper pace of the exercise by counting its cadence. Counting cadence properly was critical, because maximum benefit could only be derived from an exercise if its pace was correct.

For the leader, it was a challenge to call cadence well. First, he had to get the rhythm right. Then, he had to be able to maintain the cadence while he himself was running out of breath from performing the exercise. That was a key point about Army PT that made it different from a civilian exercise class or a sports team. The man leading PT didn't just stand there with a clipboard. He had to lead by doing everything he asked the men to do. If he couldn't do it, then he couldn't ask them to do it. So, if anything, the leader had to be in a little better shape then the men he was leading. Otherwise, he couldn't call the cadence.

The Army has a certain and well-used three-part teaching methodology for the transference of a skill. First, there is always an Explanation of what is being taught. The instructor tells the student what he will learn, why it's important to learn it, and how it will be taught. Second, there is a Demonstration of the skill that is being taught. The purpose of the Demonstration is to give the student a visual image of what the Explanation looks like in action. The instructor either demonstrates it himself, or calls upon a demonstrator to help him do it.

The Explanation (if done well) provides the student with an abstract but clear idea of what he is going to learn and how he will learn it. The Demonstration (if done well) provides him with the assurance that the skill the Explanation described to him can actually be performed because he is shown a man who can do it. However, the Demonstration does not provide the student with the confidence that he can perform the skill. For that, there is the third step in the Army teaching methodology: the Practical Exercise.

Whereas the Explanation and Demonstration focus upon the instructor through his words and actions, the Practical Exercise focuses on the student through his efforts to put what he has heard and seen into action for himself. Whereas the instructor applies a

The Solution

PART 3

one-size-fits-all approach to the Explanation and Demonstration, during the Practical Exercise he assists, corrects, and motivates each student individually, at a pace and manner that is dictated by the individual student's ability to grasp the concept and do it for himself. Thus, the instructor may have to encourage one man and reprimand another, even though there is no discernible difference in their performance at the moment. It all depends on the man and what works best for him. That is the instructor's job during the Practical Exercise.

The Practical Exercise (even if done well) will leave each student with only a working knowledge of the skill being taught. In other words, he will not be an expert but he will be able to get it done. That is how the Army transfers skills from the more experienced soldier to the inexperienced soldier. It provides formal training to get the basic skill across. After that, it's up to each soldier to improve toward mastery as he performs the skill on the job, and as he seeks to meet the increasingly high standards set for him by his leaders. Thus, an infantryman with some experience who is performing a task at minimal skill level might hear from his sergeant that he "isn't in basic training anymore." In other words, more is expected of you now. You have to improve. It's an individual soldier's responsibility to seek constant improvement. It's the leader's responsibility to demand that he do so.

So, when Dredd was taught to lead PT, he first received the Explanation and the Demonstration. He understood what he was supposed to do and he watched his instructor do it, very smoothly and with great expertise. There were thirty men in the class, so the Practical Exercise was to be spread out over time. Each man would get multiple chances to lead the rest of the class in PT. Dredd's first turn was tenth, so he got to watch nine men do it before his turn came. He wasn't worried. In fact, he was a little cocky. He was smart. He was a good athlete and in decent shape. He was a college graduate. He thought he would do at least as well as the nine men who preceded him.

Nonetheless, he didn't sleep the night before his turn came. He stayed up, making sure he had all the commands memorized and practicing the exercises until he could do them at the right cadence. By morning, he knew he had it down. So he was pretty surprised when he stepped in front of the class and forgot nearly everything he was sure he had learned. He would still be standing there today if the instructor had not prompted him, like a director to an actor with stage fright.

Once he got moving, Dredd stumbled through the formation commands, at least the half he could remember. Although he had done it perfectly in front of his bathroom mirror the night before, it was a different animal altogether with men (other than himself) looking back at him.

And that was just to get the men into PT Formation. Once there, he really began to screw up. He forgot the names of the exercises. His cadence was so far off that the men just went at their own individual paces. There was no point in trying to keep to his staccato tempo. The worst part was that he ran out of steam before he could get to the end of each exercise. That meant that he was silent (except for the sucking sounds) during the last few repetitions of each exercise. By the end, Dredd was drenched in sweat, but not from the PT. It was flop sweat. His leadership had been horrible. There was no other word for it.

An important part of every Practical Exercise is the Critique, during which the instructor tells the student what he has done well, done wrong, and how he can improve. Even though the Critique is generally focused on one man, it is usually done as a group so that all of the students can benefit. Dredd expected his Critique to be very long and embarrassing. There were so many things he had done wrong, he figured it might take an hour, but he was wrong. It took five seconds.

All the instructor said was, "Lieutenant, if we had a Museum of Failure here at Fort Benning, that performance would have its own wing." That was the entire Critique. He didn't point out

The Solution

PART 3

a single specific thing Dredd had done well (probably because there weren't any) or a single thing he had done wrong (probably because there were too many to know where to start). Anyway, the truth was that Dredd knew exactly what he had done wrong. He didn't need it spelled out for him by the instructor. He had failed to obtain even a minimal working knowledge of how to lead PT, so he should not have been surprised by the only other thing the instructor said during the Critique: "Try it again tomorrow."

Great, he thought, now I have to stink up the place two days in a row. It wasn't enough that I stayed up all night the first time and still couldn't get it right. Now, I have to do it again. And he did. He stayed up all night working on the commands and practicing the exercises. It paid off a little. The next morning he was exhausted, but he wasn't as nervous as he had been the previous day. Having failed so miserably the first time, he (and everybody else) knew he had nowhere to go but up. And he went up, a little. He didn't need the instructor's prompting to get moving and he remembered more (but not much more) than half of the commands. He was able to get to the end of some of the exercises before he petered out. At the end, Dredd had a little less sweat from flop and a little more from exercise than he had the day before.

Like the day before, the Critique was short. "Lieutenant," the instructor said, "when the circus comes to town, I'll give them your name. They are always looking for a new act. But, I'll give you this. You were better than yesterday. Not a lot better. But better."

A few weeks later, Dredd got his third chance to lead PT. This time the Critique lasted fifteen minutes. "It was," the instructor said, "marginally acceptable in parts. Other parts reminded me of the scene in *The Exorcist* when Linda Blair's head spins around."

The tenth or so time Dredd led PT, all the Instructor said was, "Congratulations, Lieutenant, you've graduated to minimal competence. Not good. But getting you to good isn't my job. It's your job to get yourself to good."

It took about a hundred PT leads for Dredd to get to good. By then, he'd left Fort Benning and was an actual platoon leader. Now, there was no instructor to critique him. He had to do that for himself. He also had to set the standard for his subordinate leaders and critique them as well. He found that he could not do that in good conscience unless he kept working towards mastery. So he did. Slowly.

By the thousandth time Dredd led PT, he had forgotten about the Museum of Failure and the goal of getting to good. He was good. By the ten-thousandth time, he could lead PT drunk, or in his sleep, or both. He could even talk and make jokes during his cadence. He was so far past good that he could start using his imagination to make PT both hard and fun. He found that by making it fun, his men didn't even seem to notice how hard it was until it was over. It was hard enough to be play. Instead of dreading it, his men looked forward to it. That, Dredd supposed in retrospect, was leadership. It had only taken ten thousand hours to get there from the Museum of Failure.

He knew that, but he didn't really think about it until years later, when he read *Outliers* by Malcolm Gladwell. Gladwell's idea is that the most important component of mastery (in anything) is practice, not the lucky accident of birth. This is *contra* conventional wisdom, but all you have to do (*per* Gladwell) to confirm its truth is look at examples of exploited and unexploited genius to see that it is so. The difference between the two is practice, lots of practice.

Mastery of anything, whether it's playing the cello or making a cheeseburger, is primarily driven by the willingness of the man seeking it to put in the required number of hours to get there. For Gladwell, that number is ten thousand. We think that this is about right.

At Fort Benning, Dredd's instructor had given him the working knowledge he needed to lead PT with minimal competence. He had also inspired him with the desire to put in the time necessary to get to good. But it was circumstances (mainly that he stayed

92

in the Army for nine years) that led him to ten thousand hours of practice. It can be a long road out of the Museum of Failure, and it is up to each man to decide how far he is willing to travel. However, it is the Q who inspires him not to be satisfied and stop along the way.

⭘ HTC

In its Q-System, F3 uses a highly modified version of the Army PT System to teach Qs how to lead a Workout. The Q still has to call the cadence, but we cut the number of commands down by about 90%. We call this system "HTC," which stands for How To Count. We don't require a Q to use HTC. He is free to lead his Workout in any way he sees fit. But he has to lead it. He cannot Clipboard and he cannot peter out. As we said before, the unwritten rule is, "If you can't do it, don't Q it." The reason we don't have to write that down is that the PAX demand it. They will not let a Q be a Clipboarder.

So, F3 being a Starfish, a Q can use any system he wants as long as he leads it.

For example, the Q can call out an exercise by OYO, which means giving the PAX a set number of a certain exercise to do "on your own." He could also just run the PAX up and down a parking deck for an hour, if that's how the spirit moves him. However, we do encourage Qs to use HTC, because we have found that it gives them confidence in their ability to lead the PAX and the opportunity to demonstrate their competence in that ability. We believe that confidence and competence are leadership building blocks, which is at the heart of F3's Purpose. In addition, HTC is interactive, so it creates esprit de corps within the PAX of the Workout. Happy workouts are magnetic, and that is the point of the First F.

These are all good reasons to use HTC in F3, but none is the most important reason, which is that HTC gives the Qs a hard objective standard against which they (and the sub-Qs they are training) can improve. HTC is hard to do, so excellence in doing it is hard to attain. Remember Tom Sawyer's Great Law of human action. Only those things that are hard to attain are both play (rather than work) and coveted by men (rather than avoided). This is the primary reason we teach HTC and encourage its use in F3 by the Qs. The hard work required to move out of the Museum of Failure provides purpose and drive to the Qs and makes working out in the Gloom a form of play rather than work. It's that simple.

Although HTC is hard to do well, F3 makes the steps simple. It is a series of three two-part commands, each of which leads to an action of sorts. In between each two-part command there is a brief pause. Here is the Explanation of what it should look like:

	PART I	PART II	ACTION
1ST COMMAND:	THE NEXT EXERCISE IS (PAUSE)	THE SIDE STRADDLE HOP!	MENTAL PREP
2ND COMMAND:	STARTING POSITION (PAUSE)	MOVE!	ASSUME START POSITION FOR EXERCISE
3RD COMMAND:	IN CADENCE (PAUSE)	EXERCISE!	BEGIN FIRST MOVEMENT OF EXERCISE

After the Q calls "Exercise" the PAX make the exercise's first movement, which the Q calls as "one," followed by the second ("two") and the third ("three"). Instead of calling "four" on the last movement, the Q is silent and the PAX call "one" — as in one repetition. The Q's call of one, two, and three is the cadence. The next time around (i.e., after the Q's "three"), the PAX call "two." On the last repetition of the exercise, the Q raises the volume and changes the inflection of his cadence. This tells the PAX that this repetition is the last, after which instead of calling a number, they call out "Halt!" The PAX remain in the halt position (the original

The Solution

PART 3

starting position) until the Q calls "Recover!" On recover, the PAX return to the standing position.

That is the Explanation. You will probably have to read that out loud a few dozen times to get the idea. To see the Demonstration you will need to go the F3Nation.com website. We posted it there for that purpose. Watch the Demonstration a few times. Then you'll only need ten thousand hours of Practical Exercise. F3 can't do that part for you, Brother. That part is up to you.

CHAPTER 3

THE GLUE OF THE SECOND F

THE FIRST F FILLS the Pogo40 hole of the Bowling Ball Grip. The Second F fills the second hole, The Sifter. Inevitably, the world will shake a man. When that happens, the damage done to the foundation of his life will depend upon the depth of his male friendships. The stronger and more stubborn his friendships are, the less likely they are to fall through the bottom of The Sifter. It's these sticky friendships that a SadClown lacks. His friendships are finite and situational. With F3, that changes. Having gotten in shape through shared pain and sweat, he finds he has formed deep bonds with the men in his Workout. When the world starts shaking, these guys don't fall out the bottom.

○ REGIONS AND NOMADS

The sticky relationships formed through F3 Fellowship are why we call the Second F The Glue. It is what makes men stick to F3. Earlier we described how clueless we were about how to get a man to plant a new Workout, but the imperative of avoiding DRTF (Diminishing Returns To Fellowship) compelled us to keep trying. The First F is the magnet of F3, but that only brings the men in. What keeps them there, what turns them into PAX, is the Fellowship, the Second F. This is The Glue. DRTF erodes The Glue, so it has to be battled.

We found that DRTF sets in at about eighteen PAX. So, we encourage bifurcation when a Workout starts rising consistently through the mid twenties to thirties. We find that splitting a thirty-man Workout does not produce two fifteen-man Workouts. It produces two more thirty-man Workouts. As noted earlier, we call this ABD (Addition By Division). We are not entirely sure why ADB works, but like a dog looking at a ceiling fan, we are just happy it does and committed to staying in the breeze.

When we figured out I2 and Mean Mean Stride, we started having success with the Q-System to plant new Workouts. That was great, but it gave us a new challenge. How to organize them all into the F3 Starfish? Were we in the small center (what we came to call F3Nation), capable of interfacing with ten, twenty, or a hundred individual Workout/appendages? We tried that for a time and found it to be chaos – the equivalent of the DRTF in a Problematic Workout, but at an F3Nation-wide level.

We saw that F3Nation needed some (limited) structure to the Starfish to be able to serve the Workout Qs properly. We needed to limit the amount of Qs with whom we had constant contact to a number that would not overwhelm us.

Napoleonic road-builders that we are, we turned to the military for an idea. The military is surely not a Starfish. Generals/admirals are on top and privates/seamen are on the bottom. In between there is a pyramidal rank structure. However, while not a Starfish, it's not really a Spider either, because the elimination of the head does not kill the body. Generals, captains, and sergeants get killed, retire (or just move on) all the time. The reason their departures don't destroy their units is that part of their job is to train their subordinates to take their place in that eventuality. Thus, if the captain commanding an infantry company is killed, the highest-ranking lieutenant automatically assumes command. If the captain was doing his job, his successor: 1) knows how to do what the captain knew how to do, 2) has a clear vision of the mission, and 3) has been encouraged to take charge by the captain who has rewarded every instance of initiative the younger man has taken.

No captain (or any other leader) can properly instill I2 in a hundred lieutenants, maybe not even in ten men. That is why the military has a span of control baked into its leadership structure. The span of control is the number of men a man can lead and influence if he is doing it properly. Generally, that number is four or five. After some study, we decided to adapt the military's model of span of control to the Starfish structure of F3. We grouped geographically-related Workouts into Regions, each headed by a Regional Q, or what we call the "Regional Nant'an."

We borrowed the Nant'an idea from the Apache Indians, as described in *The Starfish and the Spider*. A Nant'an is the unique type of tribal chief of the Apache Indians. For centuries during the era of the Spanish conquistadors and later during the United States's westward expansion, the Apaches were the one group of natives who were able to hold off all conquerors. The difference between the Apaches and the Incas or the Aztecs, the Cherokee or the Sioux, was in how they decentralized political power within the tribe.

In other cases, the Americans and Spanish were able to overcome tribes by killing or corrupting their chiefs. That model did not work with the Apache. Every time the would-be conquerors thought they had the right man, another man would pop up to lead the Apaches' stubborn and continued resistance. The Apache were not a Spider that could be killed by cutting off its head. They were a Starfish, comprised of self-sustaining appendages that were loosely connected through a cultural and spiritual leader, the Nant'an.

"The strategy failed," we are told in *The Starfish and the Spider*, "because no one person was essential to the overall well-being of Apache society."

The Apache Nant'an could not compel the Apache appendage/tribes to go to war, or anything else. He had to lead through vision and persuasion. If the appendages did not share his vision, and/ or were not persuaded to follow it, they just didn't. Thus, it did not matter if this man were killed or corrupted, another Nant'an would simply take his place.

Each F3 Region is organized in the same way. F3Nation has a Nant'an, but he is only the cultural and spiritual leader of F3. He is small. He has no power to compel a Workout Q or Regional Nant'an to do anything, with a single exception. F3Nation can cut an appendage off if it will not adhere to the F3 Core Principles. In a way, that would be like the Apache Nant'an telling a distant tribe that they weren't Apache anymore, because they weren't adhering to Apache principles. If the Nant'an didn't do that, he would run the risk that other tribes within Apache Nation would begin to be influenced or affected by the rogue group. If left unchecked, that could spread until there was no Apache Nation.

In a sense, that is what ultimately happened. The U.S. Army eventually realized there was no chief of the Apache to corrupt, so they gave the Nant'ans cows. The power held by the Nant'ans shifted from symbolic to material; they now had the power to reward and punish tribe members and they began fighting among themselves about resource allocation and other material concerns. The power structure became hierarchical and, in short order, the Apaches ceased to exist. That may be the only way to kill a Starfish organization. Make each man care about himself more than he does the organization or the other men in it. In other words, make it acceptable for each man to put himself first. Do that and the organization disintegrates into its component parts. It ceases to exist.

Each F3 Region is comprised of multiple Workouts under the loose grouping of the Regional Nant'an, who is free to run his Region as he sees fit for the benefit of its PAX. His only guardrails are the Core Principles. The Regions have the great majority of the power and responsibility within F3. The success of the Region is the responsibility of the Regional Nant'an.

To help them achieve that success, F3Nation provides support, advice, and connection to F3Nation.com. That is F3Nation's responsibility. Taking the Explanation described in the first chapter of this book and turning it into this book is part of that job. We did it to help the Regional Nant'ans plant, serve, and grow more men's small leadership groups. We did that to help them accomplish F3's Mission to reinvigorate male community leadership.

We also did it to help the Nomads, which are groups that are too small to be Regions, and too distant in geography or culture to be part of an existing Region. By geography, we mean reasonable driving distance. A Workout that takes more than an hour to reach is probably too far away for the Regional Nant'an to serve. Likewise, a Workout comprised of men who do not share the same cultural values (as opposed to F3 values as promulgated by the Core Principles) is too distinct for the Regional Nant'an to lead well. The Nomads are no less a part of F3 than the Regional Workouts, and F3Nation spends as much time and energy helping them grow (into Regions, hopefully) as it does with the Regions.

Thus, F3's organization cannot be called a true Starfish. There are certainly elements of the Starfish model we have used, but it is strongly influenced by what we have observed working in the military. As Napoleonic road-builders, we are far more interested in the evolution of what works than we are in being at the head of a revolution. Our Mission is to win the war against SadClown Syndrome. We will use anything at our disposal to get that done.

○ THE COFFEETERIA, THE HDHH, AND THE CONVERGENCE

It is the responsibility of the Workout Qs and Regional Nant'ans to find the stickiest glue available to strengthen their Fellowship. The methods they employ reflect the composition of their groups. F3Nation does not dictate or prohibit any Second F gathering (so long as it does not violate the Core Principles). However, across the Regions, there are three types of gathering that enjoy particular popularity: the Coffeeteria, the HDHH, and the Convergence.

The Coffeeteria has its roots in the Campos. After each Saturday workout session, the men who could would gather in a Caribou Coffee about a half-mile away. The only point of this gathering was to drink coffee and spend a little more time together before returning to the life of a father/husband. When we planted the Mothership, we took the idea with us and named it the Coffeeteria. Most Saturday Workouts continue the tradition, with some adding breakfast to the coffee.

HDHH stands for Hump Day Happy Hour, and means exactly what it sounds like, PAX meeting to drink beer on Wednesday night. As with the Coffeeteria, there is nothing revolutionary about the idea. It gives the PAX a chance to talk without the distraction of calling cadence or panting from the Workout. And, of course, some of us like beer.

A Convergence occurs when a Regional Nant'an combines several Workouts into a mega-workout for a holiday or other special occasion. Independence Day is a great time for a Convergence, particularly when it does not fall on a Saturday. A Convergence can also be used to gather around one of the PAX who is sick or to support another area event. We have testimonials too numerous to count of the uplifting effect on a man of seeing a cluster of F3 shirts surrounding him when he is most in need of support. It doesn't stop The Sifter from shaking, but it keeps a man upright until it stops, as it always does. Nothing (good or bad) lasts forever. That's the nature of time.

○ CSAUP

A CSAUP is any Second F gathering that is Completely Stupid And Utterly Pointless. In F3 we do a lot of that kind of thing. It's the CSAUP things that cause our wives/significant others to shake their heads and say, "I don't get it, but it seems to be working for you. So, go on." It's hard to recall exactly when these things started, but it probably traces back to the Campos's participation in the Marine Corps Mud Run near Columbia, South Carolina.

The Mud Run is an obstacle race (through the mud, obviously) in a cow pasture. It takes place twice a year, in the spring and fall. Four-person teams race against time over a thirty-six obstacle, five-mile course. About half of the obstacles involve a mud pit of some kind. The Mud Run is a completely stupid thing to do. There is no point to it, other than it is fun. It is so much idiotic fun that we kept doing it after the Mothership was planted. Every time we did it, we would get more guys who heard about it and wanted to do it with us.

It wasn't long before the Mud Run wasn't the only idiotic thing F3 did. This was in the early days of F3, before there was much of explanation for anything we did or didn't do. We would sometimes get stuck when we tried to explain this to FNGs, not so much on the "why" or the "what," but on the "why the what." That is, why we chose to do one what over another. Why, for example, the Mud Run, rather than something else?

We never had a great answer to that kind of question, until OBT came up with the CSAUP concept. CSAUP was born during the planning of what we would eventually call the GOAT. One year there was a gap between Second F events. The gap seemed too long without something to keep the PAX's energy and enthusiasm spiked. Because there did not seem to be anything good (as in bad) out there for which somebody else was responsible, we decided that we had to invent something and run it ourselves. But what? Everything we thought of required either logistical support or expertise we lacked, or was too similar to what we were already doing.

We had to brainstorm a bit. Eventually, OBT recalled the image of our man The Colonel slipping repeatedly on the muddy trail during another obstacle race. The Colonel was wearing those little feet-glove things on his tiny man-hooves (The Colonel has small feet, but a big heart) and they just would not give him enough traction to stay upright very long. Every time he fell, he looked to OBT like a middle aged Satyr with an inner-ear malfunction.

Some woman, after being knocked down by The Colonel for the third time, finally lost her temper and yelled, "That is the most irresponsible footwear decision I have ever seen for an event like this!" The Colonel just bleated at her and galloped off. OBT (running a bit behind The Colonel for safety purposes) heard the angry woman's reprimand and had to agree. He thought that it did seem kind of stupid and pointless to wear foot-gloves to a muddy obstacle race. It was irresponsible and just like The Colonel to do it anyway (one of the many reasons that we love him).

Eventually, OBT's recollection would lead to an inspiration. The F3 mid-term event needed to be something as stupid, pointless, and irresponsible as the The Colonel's footwear decisions generally were. In fact, it had to be Completely Stupid And Utterly Pointless. Once we got that far, it wasn't hard to come up with the idea of running from each Workout location in what would become the F3Metro Region (about twelve miles total) and doing a mini-bootcamp at each one. And of course, it had to be named in honor of the scruffy, irresponsible goat-like man who inspired it with his stubborn and reckless hoof-wear choice. So we called it the "GOAT," and the CSAUP concept was born.

To make sure we could do it, we tested the course by running it by ourselves first. That was prudent, but only to an extent, because we neglected to include the mini-bootcamps, assuming them to be kind of a break from the run. It didn't seem that hard to us at the time. Bad planning. About halfway through the real thing we realized the GOAT was very hard. Way too hard. It was irresponsible. Of course the Qs who led each mini-bootcamp all wanted to prove they were the biggest, baddest F3 Qs in Charlotte, and each used their ten minutes to completely smoke the PAX. By the ten-mile mark we felt like we had run twenty miles. We made the executive decision to cut off two miles and one mini-bootcamp. As it was, we had stragglers strung out for a mile or so.

The GOAT was so hard, so completely stupid and utterly pointless that … the PAX loved it. The Raleigh Region picked up the idea and did one they called The Mule. The Charlotte North Region followed up with The Bear. Workouts and Regions continue to run the Mud Run, Spartan Races, Tough Mudders, GORUCKs, marathons (sometimes without actually training), and anything else CSAUP. It's a Second F fixture.

○ THE MAGICAL GLUE OF CSAUP

Years before he and Dredd started F3, back when he was still a SadClown, OBT attempted his first CSAUP. He was 30 years old and a reporter at *The Charlotte Observer* in 2001, when he pulled together a team for a long-distance relay race in western North Carolina that was called Mountain Madness.

Twelve-person teams would launch from Asheville on a Saturday morning and run in sequence all through the day and night and into Sunday to finish in Boone. OBT had run a number of marathons and was excited to try something new — and running up and down the Blue Ridge Mountains seemed like an adventure. But he needed a team and had only been living in Charlotte for a little over a year.

Not knowing where to turn, he recruited Work Buddies. The paper's healthcare reporter signed on; so did a young woman in the design department. A metro editor and one of his friends, an assistant business editor. The paper's lead political reporter. Someone knew a guy who worked at the *Charlotte Business Journal* and was a runner, so they grabbed him. A female photographer for the paper also liked to run, so she was recruited.

Getting this motley crew to the start line felt like herding cats. One woman quit the team because her boyfriend was worried about her running through the mountains in the middle of the night. Her replacement was a young woman who was game but ran fourteen-minute miles.

The team arrived for the start of the race at 8 a.m. on a beautiful September Saturday and set off; the first runner's leg was on the Blue Ridge Parkway. The rest of the team drove ahead to the first exchange, five miles up the parkway, where they parked the SUV and got out to wait.

OBT was already worried about the team meeting the minimum twelve-minute-per-mile pace required to keep from getting pulled off the course by the race organizers. "I don't care how slow we go," he said to his friend the healthcare reporter. "All that matters is that we finish."

The metro editor and his buddy the assistant business editor were standing nearby. The metro editor shrugged: "If we fall too far behind or it stops being fun, we'll just drop out. Finishing doesn't matter."

OBT and the healthcare writer exchanged a glance, realizing this might be headed the wrong way.

As they ran up and down the mountains, race organizers warned they were falling behind the other teams. Spirits were OK until the wee hours of the morning, when members of OBT's team started started to complain and talk about quitting. As the team ran deep into a forest, with hunters' campfires visible through the trees on a moonless night, energy ebbed.

Just before dawn, the Li'l Debbie bearclaws and Donut Stix ran out inside the SUV. Ten of the team members (all except OBT and his friend the healthcare reporter) mutinied to stop for breakfast and quit the race. The team drove back to Charlotte in silence.

CSAUPs are really just are a concentrated version of The Sifter. Under the stress of the Mountain Madness CSAUP, most of OBT's teammates — all classic Work Buddies — fell out the bottom of the Sifter. Only the healthcare reporter was a sticky friend; he and OBT would continue to be close and would run several marathons together over the next few years, even after they moved on to other jobs.

Done in the context of F3 (where the assumption is that no man will fall out the bottom of The Sifter) CSAUPs are something different – something we do not in spite of their difficulty, stupidity, and pointlessness, but because of those things. After each CSAUP, there is always great emotion, fatigue, and (the point of it all) massive Fellowship. Without exception, CSAUP = Glue.

The world is probably divided up roughly between those men who seek things CSAUP, and those that avoid them for the very same reasons, because they are stupid and pointless. If you are reading this and see yourself in the latter camp, you are not wrong or crazy. You agree with our wives/significant others, and they are both smart and sane.

However, we will point out that (in our limited and unscientific observation) men who do things CSAUP (as illogical as those things are) often also end up being the guys who accomplish things, even though what they accomplish is not always what they set out to do.

Take Christopher Columbus. His logical friends probably turned down the chance to go with him in search of a backside passage to India. They probably tried to talk him out of it too. They probably told him he would sail off the end of the Earth, which was the conventional wisdom of the time. When Columbus set sail anyway, his logical friends were likely very smug, right up until the moment they heard that Columbus had discovered the New World. At that point, they probably forgot what Columbus originally set out to do and started yelling, "You wonderful bastard, you discovered another continent! We knew you had it in you." Then they wished that they had sailed with him too, no matter how CSAUP the whole adventure had appeared to them beforehand.

By then, as it always is after the fact, it was too late. That CSAUP ship had sailed. The best way to find out if a man is like Columbus or one of his logical friends is to simply tell him not to get on the boat. That's the F3 CSAUP EH method. Just tell the man about the idiotic thing you are getting ready to do. Then tell him it is really hard, that it's completely stupid and utterly pointless. Then tell him you don't think he should do it. Just say, "I'm doing it, but I don't think you should. It would be better if you didn't do it."

If he's a logical friend, he'll agree. And stay home. If he's a Columbus, he'll yank the application form right out of your hand before you can say another word. He's getting on that boat with you. He may try to take your spot. By the time it's all over, he'll be another large particle friend who won't fall out your Sifter no matter how hard the world shakes it. He's the kind of man who will be sticky. Very sticky.

CHAPTER 4

THE DYNAMITE OF THE THIRD F

THE THIRD F FILLS the last hole of the Bowling Ball Grip, purposelessness—what we call The Reacher. After a man is fit and has engaged the power of deep male friendship, we find his attention naturally turns to his hard-wired desire to serve. He finds that he wants to accomplish something that will benefit someone other than himself. That's why we define Faith (as simply as we can) as a belief in something outside of oneself.

Faith is a tricky word for us. When our Campos friend Zoot came up with the name "F3," for what we were doing at the Mothership we knew the Third F would cause some confusion, so we tried to come up with another word for it. Ultimately, after we eliminated every other possibility, Faith is what we had left. No word defines the Third F any better.

However, to be clear, the Third F has nothing to do with religion. Some of us go to church, others to temple, others don't worship in any organized fashion, but none of us is a theologian. All we are doing is recording our observation of what happens in the life of a man in whom the Third F is stirred. To us, it looks like Faith, as in a belief in something unseen and outside of the man himself.

Inevitably and periodically, we get questions about the Third F from opposing ends of a particular spectrum. One end asks us why we are so wishy-washy about our beliefs. Since many of us are

Christians, shouldn't F3 be demonstrably Christian? Shouldn't the Third F actually be a "C"? From the other end, there is skepticism about F3's agnosticism. "C'mon, stop being so tricky," these guys say. "Isn't this just another Promise Keepers or something? Shouldn't you just be honest and admit that this is a religious group?"

Essentially, both ends of this spectrum are asking for the same redefinition of Faith, but for very different reasons. One end seems intent on using F3 to evangelize, and the other end wants it branded evangelistic so it can put F3 on a list of things to be avoided. Our response to both is the same. F3's Mission is what it is. We are not out to make more of any particular letter on the COEXIST bumper sticker. F3's Mission is the reinvigoration of male community leadership. If that works, we don't care if the man is a Christian or a Druid. We have done what we set out to do.

Then, one might ask, why not do away entirely with the Third F? Why not take Faith out of the equation? Two reasons. First, you can't do away with something that clearly exists for the sole purpose of avoiding an argument. The Third F exists. Fit and friended men turn outward. They become driven. They look for like-minded men with whom they can lock shields for righteous purpose. How can we pretend that something we can see right in front of us does not exist? To deny it would make us liars.

Secondly, as we set out in the first chapter, Faith is the dynamite of F3. The outward-turning-man is what makes F3 a dynamic force in the lives of other men. It is why F3 is growing and spreading. Denying its existence would be suppression (if it were possible) of the very thing that is driving us forward. It would be like Toyota denying the existence of gasoline. That's not CSAUP, it's just stupid.

Now, and finally, the fact that F3 does not promote a particular worldview does not mean that we try to stop any F3 member from living his out. Why would we? That is why we are happy to see men (who are moved to do so) start Third F groups to study their individual faith more deeply. Any other man who wants to is free to join him, or not. We see this in the same way we see the First F. Not every man in F3 enjoys cycling. Some men (no names will be mentioned) are downright hostile to it. But that (one man's hostility) does not mean that we will keep the men who love it from having an F3/Gears group and cycling together every day if they want to. What it means is that the hostile guy is free not to join them.

The Second Core Principle is that F3 must be open to all men. We aim to stand by that.

F3 Lingo (cont.)

Counterama: *The process by which the PAX count off in the COT so that the group may know how many attended the workout.*

Namerama: *The process in which PAX in a COT announce their birth name, their F3 name, and their age.*

The Shout Out: *The brief prayer that closes every COT.*

Ball of Man: *A Shout Out formation, adopted by many F3 workouts groups, in which the PAX gather tightly around the man delivering the Shout Out, placing hands on one another.*

○ LIVING THIRD

Each F3 Workout ends with what we call the Circle Of Trust, the COT. That's not just a statement, it's the fifth and final Core Principle. If you want to call yourself an F3 Workout, you have to do a COT. You can do whatever you want to do in your COT, but there are three things you must do.

First, there must be a Counterama. The first man says "one" and so on around the circle until you get to the Q sitting in the middle. We do this because keeping track of the PAX growth in the Workout is the only way to stop DRTF before it sets in. Second, there must be a Namerama. Starting with the man who counted "one" in the Counterama, each man says his Hospital Name (what it says on his birth certificate), his F3 Name and his age. If there is an FNG, the Q names him. Personally recognizing each veteran, and immediately integrating every new man is a must. There can be no anonymity in the Workout for it to prosper.

PART 3   The Solution

How "The Stupidest Idea I've Ever Heard" Became an F3 Institution

Dredd and OBT were running one Sunday morning with Mighty Mighty Owl Bait, one of the core guys from the original Mothership workout. This was shortly after the founding of the Mothership, and MMOB was concerned that the FNGs who were pouring in were not getting a chance to become known to each other. As they ran, MMOB proposed that they end each workout by sitting in a circle so that each man could say his name and become known as a member of the PAX.

Being of a type that does not suffer fools gladly, OBT is prone to violent, snap judgments and he had one on this occasion. He flashed back to his first few months at the Campos, when it took him eight weeks to figure out which of the two relatively short, somewhat squat guys out there was Q Ball and which one was El Esbelto. As far as he was concerned, figuring out who was who and becoming known yourself was part of the rite of passage. Not to mention the idea of making grown men sit in a circle, criss-cross-applesauce like a bunch of kindergartners playing duck-duck-goose ...

"That," he declared to Dredd and MMOB, "is the stupidest idea I have ever heard."

Dredd, as usual more farsighted, saw what MMOB was getting at. Here was a way to bind in the FNGs (who continued to show up week after week) at their very first workout, make them members of the group and part of the brotherhood. Calling it the "Circle Of Trust" would be a form of self-mockery, but the underlying result could be really positive. He said he thought it was worth a try.

Well, the COT quickly became such an essential part of the F3 workout that F3 men who occasionally attended other outdoor group workouts would complain that it didn't feel right when everyone just sort of wandered off at the end of the workout without any formal ending. And when it came time to codify F3Nation's five Core Principles, OBT made sure that his error in judgment was memorialized for history by including "must end with a COT" as the fifth Core Principle.

Third, a volunteer must lead the COT in a prayer. No particular prayer is prescribed or proscribed. Admittedly, most COT prayers sound Christian because (right now) that's the predominant worldview of the PAX in F3. That may change. It may not. It depends on where and how F3 grows, not on some predetermined goal. F3 is about overcoming adversity, not achieving diversity.

Originally, when we started the COT, the prayer was done from the seated position in the circle, and some Workouts still do it that way. However, over time, most have gone to the Ball of Man formation, where the PAX gather tightly around the Q in the center and place hands on each other.

We realize that not all of the PAX in the Ball of Man may share the same worldview, and that some may be uncomfortable with any form of prayer. If that is the case for you, then bowing your head respectfully while another man shares his faith (whatever that may be) is all we ask. If you are the kind of man who can't (or won't) do that, then F3 probably won't be a good fit for you. No offense taken. No offense meant.

We have heard a lot of things in the Ball of Man. It's not unusual to hear men asking for help for another man or family member who is sick or in pain. We often hear thankfulness for the day, the Big Ball (the Earth, that is) upon which we just sweated together, or even just for the very presence of one another.

One constant theme in the Ball of Man is the importance of sharpening each other, as Iron Sharpens Iron. Thus, we often seek help being better husbands, fathers, sons, uncles, bosses, and employees; all the things that men are called upon to be. The Third F is a realization that just being those things is hard enough without trying to be them without help. More than that, it is a surrender to this idea: an insistence upon going it alone is not noble; it is selfish and prideful. The people who depend upon us to be those things that a man must be are more important than we are. We are not first. If we need help (and we know we do, each of us) then we owe it to them to seek and accept help. That help is

The Solution

PART 3

the essence of the Third F. It has nothing to do with religion and everything to do with love.

We have a tradition of conducting a Ball of Man before a CSAUP event. Like most F3 traditions, this one simply appeared, evolved, and now is. Dredd was once asked by a CSAUP-Q to lead the pre-CSAUP Ball of Man. He didn't want to let the Q down, so he thought about it throughout the entire previous day. By the time he drove to where the ShovelFlag was planted for the CSAUP, he believed he knew what he was going to say.

But, on the way there, Dredd started thinking about a book that changed everything he had planned to say in the Ball of Man. The book is called *I Am Third*. It is the autobiography of former Chicago Bears running back Gale Sayers. He wrote it forty years ago, when Dredd was only a boy. It was the book that inspired the movie *Brian's Song*, which had affected Dredd deeply when he saw it as a boy. So much so, that he probably read the book because of the movie.

It was a time in Dredd's life when he was reading a lot of athletic autobiographies. His coaches, the older athletes in his little town, and the professional athletes of that era were the heroic role models of his then-faithless life. It was from them that he learned what he knew of teamwork and self-sacrifice, to put himself last for the good of the team. Times have changed since then. It is hard for us to imagine an athlete of today's era writing a book like *I Am Third*, the theme of which was this: God is First, My Friends are Second, and I am Third.

Dredd's sudden recollection of *I Am Third* led him to a pronounced change in what he planned to say in the Ball of Man. With the PAX gathered about him that night, he asked God to forge the hearts of the 53 men who were there into one, and to have them all remember that they were Third. God was First, our families and each other were Second, and we were Third.

When he was done, he thought the prayer had been an overly subdued flop. His job, what the Q had asked him to do, was to rouse and inspire the PAX, and he had failed. His sense of failure remained with him for two hours, until one of the instructors running the CSAUP — an overnight group event that simulates Special Forces training — looked down into the wheezing, groaning ball of pain that was the 53 men who had started and yelled something Dredd recalled from his own Special Forces days: "Team is First, Your Teammates are Second, and You are Third. Don't f'ng forget that! That is the only way you will get through this night. You have to be Third!"

The Instructor's words resonated with Dredd. He had said the same thing as a young leader in the Army twenty years previously, but had forgotten it until he heard it again that night. There (in the military), the team's survival was dependent upon each of its team-members placing themselves Third. Here, in F3, the Third F was about living that way. F3 was about Living Third. That was the only way to serve the Community and the people who depended upon us.

○ THE REVERSE-FLOW INCUBATOR

In Part One we wrote about a manifestation of the Third F effect that we encountered in the early days of F3. This was the tendency of a fairly new man to ask F3 to pursue outreach projects (what we call Opportunities) as a form of service. Because most of the Opportunities had little or nothing to do with working out, they became a distraction for us, until we formalized F3's Mission to direct and protect F3's efforts and its resources.

One could misconstrue this to mean that F3 is outreach-project-adverse. That is not the case at all. The men of F3 are involved in many forms of outreach. We just go about it backwards, as one would expect from an organization based upon a Starfish model. F3Nation does not centrally identify and plan projects to push down to its members as things that we believe ought to be done. Instead, it provides a platform, an incubator, for the growth of outreach ideas that germinate in the Regions and Nomads. In other words, the projects are born in the appendages. All F3Nation does is provide minimal tending to help them grow.

This arrangement emerged over time in the usual Napoleonic road-building way and progressed pretty far before we even recognized it. When we did finally see it, we did what we usually do in F3 when we see a good idea that has taken form without our input. We name it and claim it as if it had been our idea in the first place. We're Zebra Jockeys. That means we know we look more stylish on horseback, but we'll ride a zebra if it will get us to the right place.

To find a name for F3's outreach incubator, we turned to something we had seen in Chicago. One of that city's characteristics we most admire is its proximity to Lake Michigan. What other major city has people swimming 100 feet away from skyscrapers? Amazing.

When you go to Chicago, you can take a boat tour on the Chicago River. As the boat winds through the city, the tour guide describes all of the architectural wonders you can see from the river, and there are many. However, the one that inspired us was an engineering feat: the city's reversal of the Chicago River's flow in 1900.

Before its flow was reversed, the river emptied into Lake Michigan. Because it was full of Chicago's industrial pollution, the discharge of the river into the lake caused a lot of health problems. This led the city's engineers – trying to protect the lake that was Chicago's source of drinking water – to reverse the river's flow so that the lake flowed into the river instead of vice versa. One unanticipated effect was that, a century later, the water was clean enough for swimming.

This reverse-flow idea fit precisely into what we had recognized was going on with F3's outreach. It was a Reverse-Flow Incubator. The Third F effect motivated men to toss out Opportunities, all of which were good but most of which did not directly promote the Mission. That did not mean we didn't want to see them done. It was just that we (as in F3Nation) couldn't do them and still pursue the reinvigoration of male community leadership. That alone occupied most of our meager bandwidth. After all, we were just a bunch of guys working out in a parking lot. Even now, three years after we started, we have yet to hire our first employee.

However, by adopting (after it was already working) the Reverse-Flow Incubator, we could harness the power generated by the PAX's creation and control of their own projects without having to expend any resources. All we had to do was some minor screening and then get out of the way.

The first instance of the Reverse-Flow Incubator in action was when an F3 guy was knocked for a loop by chemotherapy. His Workout buddies asked us if we thought it would be okay for them to clean his gutters and do other yardwork until he recovered. Sure, we said, that seems real solid. Go ahead.

Then another guy asked us if we would mind if he organized a clean-up and repair project at the school where his Workout planted the ShovelFlag. Of course. Knock the heck out of it.

Then some PAX told us they were going to organize an F3 after-school program for boys at a school where there weren't a lot of fathers. And so they did.

Then we heard that a couple of F3 guys were starting a mentorship program within F3. And it happened.

Then (see how this is picking up speed), before we knew it, an enterprising guy started the F3 Foundation so we could raise money to fund some of these projects (if they needed funding).

That was about the point that we called what was already happening the Reverse-Flow Incubator. We had to. The PAX had not only stopped bothering to pitch the projects to us beforehand, they had become only marginally interested in telling us about them after they were completed. We decided to declare victory and surrender. Under the Reverse-Flow Incubator, the PAX don't

The Solution

PART 3

ask or need F3Nation's participation or guidance. All they need is permission to associate their project with F3, and some space on the website to publicize it. Both of those things are free, so we don't have to worry anymore whether an Opportunity is perfectly Missional. All F3Nation needs to do is protect the F3 brand from anything that is blatantly anti-Missional. That's a pretty low bar.

> ### F3 Lingo (cont.)
>
> **OtisBomb:** *Any project that a man proposes but is not willing to lead himself. Named for people who fart on an elevator just as the door is opening, then hop out before anyone else can escape.*
>
> **Check Stroker:** *A man whose existence and impact is summed up by the simple fact that he earned some money and stroked some checks. High-earning SadClowns are often Check Strokers.*

The only other thing we require is that the man (or, now, the Region) that pitches the project also takes responsibility for its outcome. If he wants to do it, he has to be willing to Q it. With that criterion in place, we are able to strip away the OtisBombs pretty easily.

Eventually, somebody from outside of F3 observed to us that we sure had these guys organized and doing great stuff in the community. Yeah, well, that's great, but the truth is that we have not done a thing. All these projects had been invented by and come directly from F3 guys infected with the service-drive of the Third F. The PAX do the work, because it is the work they want to do rather than the work we want them to do. That's where the power comes from.

In our experience, this is exactly the opposite from the way that most community-based organizations work. Usually, programs are formulated by the organizations' leadership, who then drive them down to the members as service opportunities. Instead of a guy being free to propose a solution to a problem he really cares about, he is presented with a pre-packaged project that somebody up the food chain thinks "ought to be done."

This has happened to us repeatedly in our own church, and when it does we find that men usually have three questions: 1) How long will it take? 2) Will I get a T-shirt? 3) What if I need to quit before it's over? Can I do that, can I quit?

We don't criticize any organization for trying to get its members involved in community service. We just don't think it works very well from the top down. We think that is backwards. Instead of pushing service opportunities down, we believe an organization should help its members follow their hearts (mainly by getting out of the way). Instead of telling them what ought to be done, we believe the organization should show its members what can be done.

For organizations to change in this way, a difficult and painful cultural shift would be necessary. Men have grown accustomed to discharging their service obligations via a well-worn box presented to them, like Cub Scouts being led through a craft project.

This problem, of men passively waiting to be told what ought to be done rather than actively doing it themselves, has been creeping up on us for a long time. More than thirty years ago (1980), George W.S. Trow wrote in *The New Yorker* that "(a)n important role of a father is to give a son a sense of permission — a sense of what might be done. This still works, but since no adult is supported by the voice of the culture (which is now a childish voice), it does not work well." As a result, Trow wrote, "(i)n the absence of adults, people came to put their trust in experts."

He sums it up pretty well. The absence of male community leadership has progressively infantilized us, sapping our will toward independence and self-reliance. When we compare Trow's "sense of what might be done" to our culture's command to do what "ought to be done," we can clearly see how far into childish expert-dependence we have descended. Maybe that is why our pastors and other community leaders foist opportunities upon us. Otherwise, nothing would ever get done. Arresting this cultural devolution will require action as bold as the initiative it took to reverse the flow of the Chicago River, but we are confident that it can be done. We have seen it work in F3. Healthy men, brought together in Fellowship and finding themselves driven to serve, are more than able to do so dynamically if given the "sense of permission" cited as lacking by Trow. This, we believe, is how men are wired.

In a sense, then, the Reverse-Flow Incubator is like a permission slip. "Sure," we say, "you can do that. You can do that without us, in fact. Go ahead. Just find another guy who feels the way you do, and go get something done."

This is why we believe the Third F fills The Reacher hole. A man does not have to travel from town to town searching for something hard and purposeful to do. Nor does he have to wait for an expert to tell him what he should do. He can find what he believes needs doing right in his own Community. And he can go do it. The harder the better.

○ CONCENTRICA

Great, you may be thinking, but how do I know what needs doing in the Community? How do I come up with an idea to be incubated? There seem to be a lot of things that need doing in my Community, and also a lot of people already doing things. If I don't wait until I'm told what to do, how will I figure it out for myself? How do I have that kind of impact?

Before we get to the "how" of the impact, we need to spend some time on the "who." Who is a man supposed to impact? Everybody? We don't think so. We think that targeted impact is most effective. We believe that each man has a personal target that we call his Concentrica.

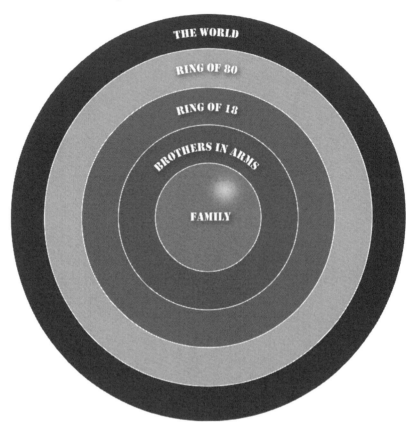

The bullseye of the Concentrica is a man's nuclear family (his wife and kids). Most of a man's impact (bad and good) will be right there. The inner ring around the bullseye is comprised of a man's closest confidants, his brothers-in-arms. Next is the ring of twelve to eighteen people (non-nuclear family, friends, and colleagues) who would be truly and deeply affected by the man's death. They would walk away from our man's funeral knowing a hole had been left in their lives by his departure from the Big Ball.

The next ring is the eighty or so people who would Post to the man's funeral and shuffle away teary-eyed (perhaps), but won't have their lives bumped far off axis by his passing. He knew them, but his impact has been far less than with the interior rings and the bullseye.

Finally, the outer ring. That is the rest of the world. The ones who won't Post to the man's funeral because they never knew him, at least not well enough to carve an hour out of their day. For this outer ring, most of us will have come and gone anonymously. But an exceptional few will actually shake things up there too. These are the men whose service to others is so profound that they have impact across their entire Concentrica. How they do that is a topic for much of the remainder of this book (and perhaps other books).

Then there is the SadClown. His passing will only be felt in the very center of his Concentrica. He is the kind of guy who has actually been fading away his entire life. With each passing day he becomes more vaporous, until he finally disappears for good with a soft, ephemeral poof. Afterwards, for a very short while, the people in his bullseye will keep his picture on the credenza, but that's about it. After that, he's gone for good. No lasting impact.

No man wants to go out that way. It's not that we don't care or aren't yearning for impact. Spend some time with retired men in Florida and you know those guys still want to matter, to be consulted, and have their opinions and experience given weight. So want-to isn't the problem. Nor is it a lack of energy and initiative. Most SadClowns expend a lot of juice with their aimless scurrying about. They talk about how tired they are. Sometimes their wives say, "Gee, the guy is always tired, but he never actually accomplishes anything with all his running around. It's pointless. What does he have to show for it?"

Tough question, but the answer is tougher: nothing. Unless we are deliberate and focused in our efforts, most of us will have little to show from our lifetime of striving. Again, not for lack of effort. The effort is there. It's the results that aren't. At most, we make some money, but in the end that just makes us Check Strokers. Not leaders. Not men of impact throughout the entire Concentrica. To do that, much more is needed. For that, a man needs a mission.

○ D2X

The Concentrica provides a man's impact target. Now we move on to identifying the arrows in his quiver. These are the things a man does to have maximum impact throughout his Concentrica. Just as we wrote F3's Mission to keep ourselves focused on solving the Problem, we believe a man must define his own personal mission to direct and protect his efforts.

This starts with what we call the D2X, or the intersection between a man's Dolphin and his Daffodil (give us just a moment and we will define these terms). That is where a man's mission is found and, if he is willing to live dangerously, where he will have maximum impact.

The importance of mission to the Third F is why so much of what F3 is and does focuses on helping men find their D2X. Without it, we are just Check Strokers with no discernible purpose other than paying the mortgage. Test this premise by asking yourself some "why" questions.

> Q: Why did I study hard in high school?
> A: To go to college.
>
> Q: Why did I go to college?
> A: To get a good job.
>
> Q: Why did I need to get a good job?
> A: To support my family.
>
> Q: Why . . . wait!! Is the answer to every why-question going to be the first part of another why-question. Where would that end? Isn't there some underlying force driving all of this, or am I just destined to be a Check Stroker who rolls over at the end and asks if his last check is going to clear?

We believe we are designed for more than that. Every man has a Dolphin (a unique and powerful skill), a Daffodil (the people of his heart's desire that he is meant to serve), and a specific Purpose

The Solution

PART 3

in doing so. We believe that these three elements comprise a man's mission, his D2X, and that the desire and I2 he brings to that mission will be defined by his willingness to live dangerously.

The Dolphin

We'll start by defining the Dolphin. Picture yourself swimming in the ocean. You may be an adequate but not great swimmer. The limits of your ability would be made very clear if an Olympic champion, say Michael Phelps, swam by you. He's been practicing all of his life. He has some physical gifts that you lack. But as good as he is, he would be like a fish out of water if a dolphin swam by you both.

Even though Michael Phelps is a great swimmer, the dolphin would swim circles around him. Like Michael, the dolphin is a mammal, not a fish. But the dolphin has fins and a blowhole. He was born not only to swim, but to spend his life in the water. It is so natural to him, and he is so good at it, that while he is swimming he has that crazy dolphin-grin on his dolphin-face and makes those crazy dolphin joy noises. In contrast, Michael Phelps is silent and grimaces with the effort he has to make. Actually, he looks a lot more like you than the dolphin looks like him.

Every man has something he does as well as the dolphin swims. Like the dolphin's ability to swim, it's the thing he was born to do. When he does this thing, his Dolphin, it's so effortless for him that it doesn't feel like work, regardless of how hard it would be for a man who had a different Dolphin. And, while he's doing his Dolphin, he is just as crazy happy as the dolphin is when he is swimming. If, by luck or design, he manages to be paid for doing his Dolphin, well then he might be leaping out of the water making crazy dolphin noises as well.

If you've read this far, you know we haven't created anything new in F3, including this thing (other than calling it the Dolphin, we did make that up). The idea of man being individually and uniquely gifted is at least two millennia old. We know this because the Bible describes it in terms of spiritual gifts. Every man has one. Thus, it's hard to explain our culture's apathy (if not hostility) toward Dolphin-finding. For some reason, in our culture, it is not unique gifts that are celebrated, it is well-roundedness – the opposite. We are not supposed to be fanatical about the one thing we really do well. We are supposed to spend valuable time doing things at which we are ill-equipped.

Men generally surrender to this cultural idea. Our man La Russa (not the retired baseball manager, but nicknamed for him) nailed the reason why when he said that there are two things that keep a man from even trying to find his Dolphin. These two things are pride and fear.

A man's pride keeps him married to some idea he has of the ideal thing he is supposed to do. Even if he can't do it. Even if he does something else very well. Still, his pride will lead him to deny it. Take the Dolphin of teaching. A man may suspect that he was born to do it, but pridefully believes that teaching is for those who can't do. Or he thinks it's for women, or pointy-headed intellectuals. So he denies it to himself. His pride keeps him from it. He would rather be miserable doing something at which he is incompetent, but which does not violate his egocentric viewpoint.

If his pride doesn't stop him from finding his Dolphin, then his fear of failure will. Once he acknowledges his Dolphin, he loses his excuse of not knowing what it is and will have to stop procrastinating and just do it. And then he might fail. It's safer to spend your life half-heartedly looking for your Dolphin that it is to find it and have to live into it.

The Daffodil

The other "D" of the D2X is the Daffodil. This is the object of a man's heartfelt desire. We use the Daffodil as a convenient image (which happens to be alliterative with Dolphin), but it actually refers to the type of person (not a particular person) that a man is hard-wired to serve with his Dolphin. We call it the Daffodil because of an experience Dredd had in the military.

In 1990, Dredd went through the Special Forces Qualification Course at Fort Bragg. It was great and thorough training to lead a Special Forces A-Team. At the time, he was an experienced captain in his fifth year of service on active duty. Before volunteering for Special Forces, he had been an Infantry officer, where he already received a lot of great leadership training and challenging assignments. So, by the time he took command of his A-Team he had about as good as possible an opportunity to know what the heck he was doing, and he thought he did.

But he didn't. There was a problem with his leadership style that only became apparent on the A-Team. He was a technically proficient leader, but his interpersonal skills were horrible. This had not been a big problem for him in the Infantry because a jerk-based leadership style was more or less accepted there. But it didn't fly in Special Forces, where persuasion was more important than direction.

The men on his A-Team were all highly competent and bold leaders in their own right. They didn't need him to tell them what to do. Sure, they would "comply" with his orders because he outranked them, but they would only truly follow him if he persuaded them to do so. Mere grudging compliance is a far cry from willing follower-ship. Dredd could see that he had to do something if he wanted to be effective.

Here is what he did. He read a book called *How to Win Friends and Influence People*. It was written by a guy named Dale Carnegie and had nothing at all to do with the military. At first, Dredd was pretty skeptical. It seemed kind of hokey to him and, as it had been published in 1936, the language was dated and off somehow. As he turned the first few pages he could feel the urge to chuck it aside and just embrace the inner jerk that he knew he was. And then he came across something in the second chapter of the book that convinced him to see it through to the end. Carnegie had Three Techniques in Handling People, and the second one was to "give honest and sincere appreciation." A leader was supposed to be "hearty in approbation and lavish in praise," especially to those who need it most.

It wasn't that particular technique that convinced him to read the rest of the book. He never praised anybody and was toughest on the very guys who needed praise the most. He thought that was what a leader did. So, that tip wasn't what got Dredd's attention. It was the story Dale Carnegie used to illustrate his point. It was about a woman named Dunham who was supervising a poorly performing janitor that the other workers mocked for his incompetence. After Dunham started to praise him for small things he did well, the janitor's overall performance improved enough that the other employees noticed it and began praising him as well. A little praise had turned the man around.

Heart-warming (and a great tip), but hard-hearted Dredd would not have cared a lick if Carnegie had not included this single detail: the story took place in the town of New Fairfield, Connecticut. In 1930, about when the book was written, the population of New Fairfield was 434 people. Sixty years later, when Dredd read the story, it had only increased to 12,911. We're talking about a really, really small place. A bump in the road with (literally) a single traffic light at the center of town. Dredd knew that because it is the town in which he was raised. There were still Dunhams there when he graduated from high school. This was years before he believed in anything outside of himself, but he must have seen some kind of karma, kismet, or kumbaya in the coincidence because he took that as a sign that he was supposed to read the whole book and at least try to do what it said. And he did.

The first of Carnegie's Six Ways to Make People Like You (the man was big on lists) was to become genuinely interested in other people. The best Dredd could do was fake genuineness, but he resolved to try. He got his first chance to do it when a new sergeant was assigned to his A-Team. He wasn't new in the sense that he had just put on the Green Beret. He was only new like a used car is new if you haven't driven it before. This guy was not bold and competent like the other sergeants on his team. He was chunky and beaten down, and he had already been passed around from team to team in the battalion. He was a marginal performer who probably should have been kicked out of Special Forces, but it was easier just to pass him off to the next team to deal with when he wore out his welcome.

As soon as the new man walked through the door, the other men on the team started rolling their eyes. Dredd's first thought was that he was going to kick this guy around for awhile until the battalion moved him to another A-Team. The same thing every other team leader had done before him. But then he remembered the janitor from New Fairfield.

So he gave it a shot. He tried to become genuinely interested in the new guy.

That didn't go so well at first. Dredd didn't exactly hold the book open as a guide while he was doing it, but he may as well have, he was so bad at it. Of course the new man didn't buy it. Dredd's efforts to talk to him about anything more than what he was supposed to do on the A-Team got nowhere. He just did the minimum to keep out of trouble and stayed in his shell.

But Dredd was (and is) stubborn, so he kept at it. One day he noticed a magazine on the new man's desk, and it was not of the usual guns, porn, and cars variety. It was about gardening.

"Hey, Sarge," Dredd said to the new man. "What's up with the gardening magazine?" The new man looked up suspiciously and made a move to put the magazine away.

"Why are you asking, sir?" he replied.

"I don't know. I just thought it was interesting. You into gardening?" Dredd asked, shooting for casualness instead of sincerity, thinking that was about as good as he could do.

"Well, yeah. I am," the new man reluctantly replied.

Dredd couldn't think of what to say next to keep this fiery conversation on track so he just asked him stupidly, "Uh . . . well, what's your favorite flower?"

Surprisingly, the new man had an answer. "The daffodil," he said. "The daffodil is my favorite."

"Why?" Dredd asked.

And then the man told him. And he told him. And he told him. Dredd figured that he had yet to get to the point of the book where Dale Carnegie gives you his Seven Tips to Politely Withdraw From a Conversation About Flowers, because all he could do was nod, smile, and hope somebody pulled a fire alarm or something. The new man's heart beat for daffodils. That was clear.

Dredd would love to say today that as a result of his taking an interest in the new man's love of daffodils that the man became a great soldier – but there are already enough Truth Nuggets in this story. What did happen is that he became a decent soldier with whom Dredd had a decent relationship. It didn't occur to Dredd until later that the new man wasn't a "slug" or a "dud" (what they called underperforming soldiers), it was that he was radically misaligned with his Dolphin. The man should have been gardening, not soldiering, and we hope that is what he is doing today (wherever he is), because if that man is growing daffodils, it's a good bet everybody around him thinks he is a freaking dynamo.

Just like the sergeant, every man has a Daffodil of his own. The hard part is figuring out what it is. But we believe that it's critical that you do so. If your Dolphin is actually gardening, it is not enough to grow any crop. You have to grow your own Daffodil (whatever it is) if you are to have dynamic impact.

Dredd encountered this truth shortly after he discovered his own Dolphin, which happens to be teaching. It was a wondrous thing to him to find his gift, so of course he initially assumed it had universal applicability. He thought he could have impact wherever he used it. So he was pretty surprised and confused to find out that this was not true. Sometimes he had dynamic impact, but other times he had far less, even though he was applying his Dolphin in the same way every time. What made that more frustrating for him was that the low-impact applications of his Dolphin exhausted him, while the times when he had dynamic impact were like rocket fuel.

The Solution

PART 3

Why was that? He thought maybe it was random or based on circumstances like the time of day that he taught or the location. But that didn't seem to correlate.

He pushed on, though, and eventually, the key factor became clear: It wasn't when or where he taught, but who he taught that made the difference. His teaching had a real effect on men – and not just any men, but men who were looking to have true impact in their lives (the sort of men who might still be reading this book …).

It wasn't that Dredd couldn't teach women or children or men who were too overcome by SadClown Syndrome to care about impact. It was that his teaching didn't have the same effect on these other groups. It was groups of maturing men who most often invited him to teach them and whose invitations he was most excited to accept. These maturing men were the ones he most wanted to serve, for whom his heart beat in the way that he had seen his gardener-sergeant's heart beat for his daffodils.

And when Dredd applied *his* Dolphin to *his* Daffodil, he found that his impact was dynamic and virtually effortless. That application, that intersection of the thing he did best with the people he loved most, was his D2X.

We now see this effect in the men of F3. They have the most impact at the intersection of their personal Dolphins and Daffodils. This is the D2X impact zone. The more a man is willing to live dangerously at that intersection, the more impact he has.

◯ PUTTING IT TOGETHER

Here (for context) is a definition of the word mission: "an important assignment carried out for political, religious, or commercial purposes, typically involving travel." This definition matches the F3 concept of Mission in the sense that it is an "important assignment" for a "purpose." We call the "important assignment" the Task; put together, the Task and the Purpose are the two components of the Mission.

Taken together, a man's Task equals his Dolphin plus his Daffodil, his D2X. So for Dredd, the Task was "to teach maturing men." His Purpose might be "to reinvigorate male community leadership."

Taken as a whole, Dredd's mission (Task + Purpose) is: *To lead and teach maturing men in order to reinvigorate male community leadership.*

Note the similarity to F3's Mission: *To establish, grow, and serve small workout groups (Dolphin) for men (Daffodil) in order to reinvigorate male community leadership (Purpose).*

Now note a couple of things about how the Missions of Dredd and F3 fit together:

1. The Purpose is the same for both. That's because Dredd serves F3 with his time. Obviously, not every man in F3 will have that Purpose.

2. Dredd's Daffodil is much narrower than F3's Daffodil. F3's service-focus is "Men," roughly one half of the population. The man's service-focus is on a very small segment of the population of Men, those who are "maturing".

3. Dredd's Dolphin reflects his individual gifts and abilities, while F3's Dolphin requires a team effort of united individual gifts.

○ PURPOSE

The second half of a man's Mission is his Purpose. Earlier, in describing how we determined F3's Mission, we referred to the Task as the What and the Purpose as the Why. A man's Purpose is also Why he does the What. The Purpose is the answer to all the "why questions" we asked before. It is where they all lead, as opposed to just another why question.

Another way to look at Purpose is that it is the solution to a man's Life Problem. There is nothing philosophical about a man's Life Problem. It's simply the thing that bugs him the most, the thing that nags at him and won't go away, unless he sets about solving it. Most men learn to live with their Life Problems, which is a big part of how they end up as SadClowns. A few men refuse to accept their Life Problems. They stubbornly set out to find a solution. If they succeed, they find their Purpose. If they pursue their Purpose with great skill and fortitude (i.e., they live dangerously), they have impact. Big impact.

To define F3's Purpose, we reverse-engineered the Problem we saw that F3 was solving. We determined it to be SadClown Syndrome. Doing it backwards like that meant that we already had the solution, which was F3. We believe that we have tested this premise long enough to know we were right. F3 is the solution to SadClown Syndrome. It fills the holes in a man's Bowling Ball Grip and gets him moving.

But we do not mean to imply that every man in F3 has SadClown Syndrome as his Life Problem. That's impossible. F3 would not be working if we tried top-down enforcement of F3's Life Problem. That, in fact, is the point of the Reverse-Flow Incubator. Instead, F3 encourages each man to discover his own Life Problem and devise a solution to it. In other words, each man works out his own Purpose. All F3 can do is help him find his own unique D2X and apply it to that Purpose in the form of a Mission.

Once a man has his Mission, he can find other men with a similar Purpose in F3. Together, they can conspire for its accomplishment. It makes sense that men with shared Purpose and complementary D2Xs would lock shields together to do battle against a shared Life Problem. We say it makes sense because it is logical and we have seen it work. But we also know that it is counter-cultural. The culture calls for well-rounded men who work outside of their comfort zones. F3 advocates the exact opposite: men who spend most of their time doing the thing they do best to serve the people they love most. We reject the concept of well-roundedness as a stultifying OprahBomb. We believe a man is made to exploit his Dolphin, not struggle to get better at the skills that comprise the Dolphins of other men. His time spent doing that would be better spent finding those guys and locking shields with them.

Likewise, we don't encourage men to get outside of their comfort zone. That too is an OprahBomb. Instead, we advocate going more deeply in. Why? Because a man is more impactful and effective inside his impact zone than anywhere else.

How does a man determine his Life Problem so he can work out his own Purpose? There is no pat formula for that either. He just has to think about his life and what has always bugged him. Take the example of Dredd again. When he left the service after nine years, he went to law school. This marked the beginning of a fifteen-year stretch of his life during which he had no definitive Purpose and no clue that he was suffering from SadClown Syndrome.

Dredd's transition from soldier to student took place over a single weekend. He left the service on Friday and started law school on Monday. Nothing in between but moving his furniture. Culture shock does not quite sum it up. It was more like being ejected unexpectedly from the front seat of your car and landing in a different decade.

The very first thing Dredd noticed that was different about law school was the lack of purpose. In the service, every man always knew his mission, his unit's mission, and the mission of the next higher unit. That meant that a man knew what he was doing and why he was doing it at all times. The next thing he noticed was the lack of leadership. In the Army, every man was both leading and being led at all times. It was an environment so infused with the call to leadership that after a while a man ceased to notice it, the way we don't notice the air we breathe until the oxygen is cut off. It was just a given that if a man had a problem to solve his boss would help him do that. In fact, he was expected to start helping before you even recognized it yourself. Another way to describe it is that it was a culture of accountability, where a man was responsible for everything that happened and failed to happen, and so was every other guy. It was hard to go off the rails. Every relationship stayed in The Sifter.

There were other ex-military guys in Dredd's law school class. About three months into that first year, one of them (a Navy man) asked Dredd if he was happy there. "No, not really," Dredd said.

"I hate this freaking place!" the Navy man retorted immediately. "I hate it! You want to know why? Because everybody here is a selfish prick and doesn't even know it."

Dredd could see what his friend meant and understood and shared his anger. There really didn't seem to be anybody in charge, and the men who should have been in charge (the professors) acted like they weren't responsible for anything. They would be late for their own classes and act as if it didn't matter. It didn't seem important to them if any of the students learned anything. It was as if their teaching and the students' learning were two disconnected elements.

One day, one of Dredd's professors left a note for him to come see him in his office. When Dredd got there, the professor asked him if he was mad at him. "No," Dredd said. "Why?"

"Well, you seem very angry," the professor replied. "I thought it might be something I said or did."

"No," Dredd replied. "I'm angry in general, I guess, but it has nothing to do with you in particular."

"Great," the professor said, looking relieved. "Thanks for stopping by." Afterward, it occurred to Dredd that the exchange was typical of the law school culture. The professor was in authority (whether he liked it or even acknowledged it) over the class, and thus

Dredd. He recognized a problem: Dredd's anger. But all he cared about was whether it was directed at him. When he determined it wasn't, his inquiry ended. What if Dredd was angry at another professor and ended up beating that guy to death with a claw hammer in the parking lot the next day? Dredd assumed that first professor would have just shrugged and said, "Oh, I guess it was old Ned that set that crazy bastard off. Interesting. Glad it wasn't me."

That professor's approach is radically different from what a leader would have done in the Army (at least the Army Dredd was in). There, if he saw a problem and didn't take reasonable steps to solve it, he would have failed even though it ultimately had nothing to do with him. That's because the focus in service was on the unit (i.e., the community), not the individual. Soldiers lived and worked with a purpose, and that purpose was the good of the unit (in general) and the accomplishment of the specific missions with which the unit was tasked. In a sense, everybody was responsible for everything. As a leader in the Army, you lived Third. Law school was totally different. It was a group of individuals parallel playing together for their own self-oriented reasons. Nobody was responsible for anything but themselves. Everybody lived First.

After Dredd graduated from law school, he realized that the lack of purpose he first observed there was not unique to that place. It was the way of the world. Every institution he encountered was just like law school, in that the men in those institutions seemed to take no responsibility for the atmosphere in which they lived and worked. They were completely inert, waiting, perhaps, for someone to tell them what they ought to do. Some expert, maybe.

Sure, there were exceptions, but only enough to prove the rule. Moreover, since those few exceptional men were isolated by the prevailing institutional culture, they had no observable impact. It was as if there was a general failure of male community leadership, and it didn't take long before it swallowed Dredd too. He quit. Disconnected from a leadership culture, Dredd became just as inert, aimless, and irresponsible as every other SadClown

The Solution

PART 3

he encountered. He steadily regressed as a man during that fifteen-year stretch, to the point where he too lived First.

Earlier, we told you that we are not social scientists, and that this book is not about why or how the decline of male community leadership came about. It might be tempting to blame somebody, but that wouldn't solve the Problem. Yet that is what Dredd did during those fifteen years in his me-first desert. He cursed the darkness instead of lighting a lamp. And it got him nowhere.

Nowhere is where he would still be, if not for F3. In that, he has found his Purpose: the reinvigoration of male community leadership. In coming together to achieve that purpose, Dredd and OBT moved along what we now call the Impact Curve. We went from SadClowns — worried about balancing needs and resources, hoping that final check would clear – to Servants, men of impact.

THE IMPACT CURVE

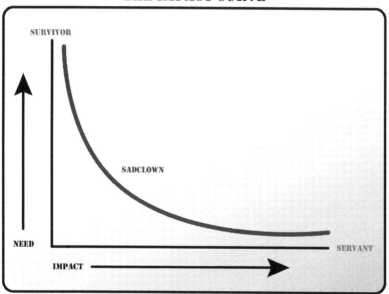

From Survivor to Sad Clown to Servant

○ THE THIRD 500

OBT's dad left his mom in 1974, when OBT was 4 years old. His mom took OBT and his younger brother and moved from Southern California to the San Francisco Bay Area, where he grew up seeing his dad for a week during the summer and another week at New Year's or winter break.

This was nothing unusual; white-collar California was Ground Zero for the divorce epidemic in the 1970s and 1980s. OBT remembers paging through his middle school and high school student directories and noting how many of his classmates listed parents with separate addresses and phone numbers.

Growing up in the Bay Area during the Joe Montana years, OBT and his brother were sports crazy, but their mom had no interest in athletics and — because she worked full time — little capacity to drive them to practices or encourage participation. Not being particularly athletic herself, she cared about academics and grades, and that was what OBT focused on. He played one desultory season of youth soccer in the fall of fifth grade, picking at the grass and staring at the sky while the game went on around him.

This was an era before anti-bullying initiatives, so OBT had been made well aware of his athletic shortcomings by the time he reached middle school. Geek, nerd, whatever you wanted to call him, there was nothing that he could do about that — but he was also on an academic track that won him a National Merit Scholarship and got him admitted to Harvard.

And it was at Harvard, in the fall of 1988, that he went to the Freshman Union, to an open call for novices interested in participating in the crew program. He got a crimson T-shirt that said "CREW '92" in giant letters across the back, and he started going to practices.

In those days, when only a handful of northeastern prep schools and scattered other schools had high school crew programs, building a freshman crew at Harvard was an attrition game. One hundred fifty novices — heavyweights and lightweights — showed up at that meeting for the free T-shirt, which they all wore as they ran around Harvard Yard to dorm parties during Freshman Week. Maybe 120 ever posted for a practice; 70 remained by the time midterms rolled around in late October. They dropped by ones and twos after that; by the time the Charles River thawed in the spring of '89, 16 novices and eight experienced oarsmen would make up the three freshman heavyweight boats that competed in spring racing.

OBT was one of them, having learned the basics of handling a sweep oar in the fall, then enduring a winter of off-the-water conditioning and technique work in the indoor tanks located on the ground floor of Newell Boathouse.

The goal in any boat larger than a single scull is to get two, four, or eight men rowing in unison, sliding forward in rhythm, dropping their oars in the water ("the catch") at the same moment, then opening with the legs, the back and, finally, the arms in synchronicity. When a crew works in rhythm, there is said to be swing in the boat — and it is this swing that moves an eight-man boat through the water with a momentum that is far greater than the sum of its oarsmen's brute individual efforts.

OBT's coach was Fred Borchelt, four years removed from rowing in the eight-man USA boat that won silver at the Los Angeles Olympics. OBT was in the tanks with Fred one Friday morning that fall, frustrated as he tried to refine the technique and motion with which he was dropping the oar in the water at the catch, when Fred said something to him that no one had ever said before.

"You know you're a natural athlete, right?"

Well, actually, no … he hadn't known that. No one had ever said anything like that to him before.

That was the first thing that Fred said to him that OBT would never forget.

The second was something that OBT would carry with him through the rest his life, that he would come to accept as one of life's core truths and that would hit him with the force of revelation one August morning in 2011, as he sat in an F3 COT.

In the spring of '89, as the freshman heavyweight crews prepared for racing season, Fred sat them down.

A head-to-head crew race was 2,000 meters long, he explained — about six to seven minutes in length, depending on conditions. For most of the race, the oarsmen would be in oxygen debt, their hearts and lungs working anaerobically to try to get energy to muscles that were drastically outworking their ability to deliver oxygen through the bloodstream.

The only way to survive, Fred told OBT and his teammates, was to divide the race into quarters — four 500-meter segments.

For the First 500, Fred told them, they would be sprinting off the line, the crew's cadence probably up around 44 strokes a minute. Full of adrenaline, they wouldn't yet be in oxygen debt. Those first 500 meters would fly by.

In the Second 500, their coxswain — the little Asian dude sitting in the bow of the boat — would get on the intercom and settle them to their race cadence, 36 strokes per minute. Now the race was joined and they would be focused on finding that swing, hitting their rhythm as a crew, coming together for the journey ahead.

The Fourth 500 — well, Fred said, that was simply "balls to the wall." Pull with anything and everything you have left. The finish line is almost here; give all that you have left, empty the tank, fight to the end … all that stuff.

It was the Third 500, Fred told them, where the race would be won or lost. That was the valley of the shadow of death. The start would be a distant memory, lost in the fog of fatigue and the buildup of lactic acid in their muscles, the finish too distant to even contemplate. If they could hold it together — as individuals and as a crew — in the Third 500, that would be the difference.

The Solution

PART 3

Fred was right. His advice proved true in that spring 1989 racing season but also, and more importantly, as OBT entered adulthood. As a senior in college, he ran his first marathon, then dozens more afterward. Always, it was Miles 13-20 — the Third 500 of the marathon — that were the toughest stretch. If he could come through that section strong, he knew he could finish well.

If you want to simulate the effect without running a marathon, go out and run a hard mile on a quarter-mile track. See if that third lap isn't the toughest.

Watch a football or basketball game. Sure, you'll get an occasional blowout that's decided within minutes of the game's start. More often though, it's the third quarter that determines the ultimate direction and outcome — a football team marches downfield on its first possession of the third quarter to tie a game that ultimately goes down to the wire; a basketball team opens the second half with a 14-2 run that blows the game open.

And sitting in a COT one August morning in 2011, as the Pax went around for the Namerama, OBT realized that F3 was also about the Third 500.

"Don Millen, Hitman, 43 … Henry Duperier, Moniteur, 43 … Jim Cotchett, Crotch Rocket, 43 …"

In the months that followed, "43" would become an F3 in-joke, but it was no joke. F3 worked because it was addressing the fundamental desire for Purpose that men have as they enter the Third 500 of their lives.

Birth to college graduation was the First 500 (bursting off the line, charged with adrenaline, 44 strokes a minute). College to 40 was a man's Second 500 (settling into a career, marriage and kids, finding your rhythm and your "race pace"). With any luck, 60 to 80 (or beyond) would be the Fourth 500, and a man would have the choice of a gentle glide path to the finish or to rage against the dying of the light.

But 40 to 60 — the time of the stereotypical midlife crisis — was the Third 500. The start line was long gone, the finish not yet in sight. Too many men were lost out here at the midpoint, wondering what they'd gotten themselves into, losing the will to drive forward, questioning why they'd come so far when the finish seemed so far away. The symptoms of the midlife crisis — the divorce, the sudden career change, the new sports car — were efforts to change external factors when the real problem lay within: Am I nothing more than a Check Stroker? Why do I feel like a SadClown? As Dredd noted, the reason F3 had such impact for these men was that they were at an age where authority collided with mortality and the question became, "What song will they sing over me when I am gone?"

For Third 500 guys, F3 is a reason to get off the Pogo40 (or, for some, off the couch entirely for the first time in years). In the Magnet of the First F and the Glue of the Second F, they find a path to Purpose, and the Third F allows them to take up the mantle of authority that they have unknowingly inherited.

What is this authority? Think about it this way: Without any notice or fanfare, a man of 43 takes stock of his life and realizes that something very important has shifted while he was busy building his career and raising his children. Things are different now. When he looks for the authority that has always been there, older and external to him, he can't find it.

Suddenly, he realizes that he is looking in the wrong place. To find authority at 43, he needs to be looking in the mirror. He is authority. And for the first time in his life, he doesn't chafe at authority, as he did when he was in his First 500, bumping up against parents, teachers, and coaches, or in his Second 500, when he recognized the need for authority figures, but viewed them as set apart from him by age and experience.

Now, he just feels naked.

The Solution

PART 3

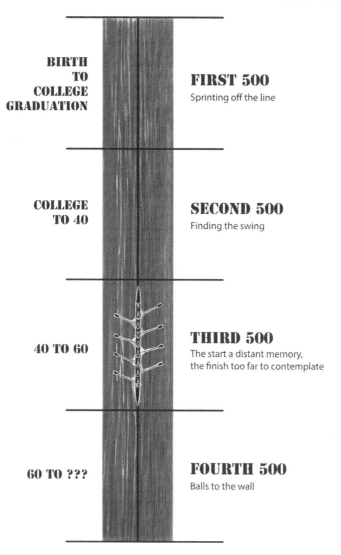

BIRTH TO COLLEGE GRADUATION	**FIRST 500** Sprinting off the line
COLLEGE TO 40	**SECOND 500** Finding the swing
40 TO 60	**THIRD 500** The start a distant memory, the finish too far to contemplate
60 TO ???	**FOURTH 500** Balls to the wall

We believe this naked feeling to have inspired that particular prayer in the Ball of Man, the one that we be made better fathers, husbands, bosses, and all other things a man has to be. It is an authority prayer or, more accurately, a request for help in discharging the obligations of authority. Part of our mild rebellion as boys and young men against authority was driven by the natural masculine desire to take the wheel and see if you can steer the ship better than the old man. By the time a man reaches 43, reality has cured him of that. By then, a man knows how heavy lies the mantle of leadership, and he is wary of the responsibility that comes along with authority. Yeah, it's your hand on the wheel of the ship, but it's also your responsibility to see that the thing doesn't sink with all the passengers on board. Those two things, authority and responsibility, they come together. You don't quite grasp that until you've hit 43, and by then it's too late to turn back.

By 43 you've made the decision in your life whether or not you will take on the responsibility that comes with authority. You know whether you've chosen to be a leader or a Mascot. If you've chosen the former, then you know you need help. That's what the prayer is about. It's a prayer for help. And the other men in the Ball of Man who are praying with you are not only asking for the same thing but implicitly promising to join with you in mutually providing it, without judgment.

Over time, as F3 grew and expanded and the viral effects of the Emotional Headlock took their natural course, the Ball of Man came to include more than just guys in their Third 500. Men in their 50s and even 60s started coming out for workouts, and one of them Reverse-Flow Incubated the idea of the CORE workout — little to no running, for guys with bad knees or just off the couch or rehabbing from injuries.

And once some of the Third 500 guys started recruiting guys who were a few years younger than themselves — younger colleagues at work, guys they knew through church or neighborhoods — Second 500 guys poured into F3. First the mid-30s guys, then the early-30s guys, then some kids in their 20s. Their fresh legs at the front of the pack and in the Q rotation cranked up the intensity of the workouts and the men themselves ate up F3, bringing all their "young, dumb, and full of ..." enthusiasm to bear on the organization.

Out of that demographic shift grew numerous informal relationships and, eventually, a formal mentoring program. Yes, it became clear, F3 was a solution (reverse-engineered, stumbled across, failed into as always …) to the Third 500 Problem, to SadClown Syndrome. But how much better for guys to never develop SadClown Syndrome, to get that swing in their boat in their 20s and 30s, and then accelerate right into and through their Third 500?

Every man in an F3 Ball of Man — whether Second, Third, or Fourth 500 — is there because he has chosen leadership over Mascot-ship by accepting the obligations of authority. And we are all in exactly the same boat. We are all idiots in the COT, that we know, but we are the idiots upon whom our communities depend to protect them from nakedness. From the COT we draw what we need to bear up to the responsibility that comes with 43, to not waver and pull our hands from the wheel at the very moment the passengers most depend upon us to keep the ship off the rocks. Without that, being a leader rather than a Mascot at 43 would be a very naked and lonely thing. It might make the SadClown life look pretty attractive. F3 helps a man resist that temptation, but not for his own sake. He is Third. He resists for those he loves. He resists for love.

○ LOCKED SHIELDS OF THE MINIVAN CENTURIONS

An axiom of military tactics is that as the lethality of weapons increases so does the distance between warriors in battle. Before gunpowder, when the primary weapons were the sword and dagger, men were tightly packed together to achieve mass and mutual protection. In addition to the blades, each man carried a shield that consisted of a heavy shank of wood bolted onto a metal boss that served as a handle. If the battle was fierce enough, the wooden part would need replacing. And it often did.

We picture that kind of soldier in an open arena using the shield to ward off blows in single combat. But that's gladiator stuff. The real purpose of the warrior's shield was as part of a wall formed in conjunction with the other soldiers in his unit. When two sides joined in battle, their leaders would call for the formation of opposing shield walls. Each warrior would lock his shield with those of the men to his left and right. It was from behind this shield wall that the armies would fight, massing their sword power together to overcome their enemy. The side whose shield wall was first broken was the side that was overcome. Break the wall, and you break the man.

The Romans were most skilled at this. Their leaders were centurions, who commanded eighty men each. It was the centurion's job to train his men and deploy them in combat. He picked the high ground to form his shield wall, called his men into it, and then exhorted them to keep it locked, to fight, survive, and win. On the strength of its skilled centurions, the Roman Army could survive and win against a determined and larger foe because in the heat of battle the centurions kept their shields locked. Break the wall, and you break the man.

And so it was until the advent of gunpowder, which rendered the wooden shield obsolete. Men still massed together to achieve superior firepower but with only their flesh and bones to act as a shield. While the Civil War found men massing in the open, World War I had them spread into trenches, and World War II spread them further into foxholes. Today, infantrymen fight as far apart as they can to protect the unit from the lethality of the enemy's weapons, but they still mass fire and still retain the emotional bond of the shield wall. For while the weapons have changed, the warrior heart has not. We still fight together, behind the shield wall, or we are overcome. Break the wall, and you break the man.

There are many great Workout locations in F3Nation, but Charlotte's Freedom Park was the first. It is where it all started. Not only is it a great place for a Workout, it also serves the community in a thousand different ways. The average man in F3Metro probably spends an average of 7 hours a week there in one capacity or another. Go there on a Saturday morning in the spring or fall and you will see the parking lots stuffed full of minivans and the fields overrun with kids playing soccer and

PART 3   The Solution

144

baseball. There is so much sweet America there it will make your teeth hurt. When the world is running particularly amok, a day in Freedom is all a man needs to keep him focused on what we have here, what is worth protecting. The World may be afire, but we have Freedom, Brothers. We have Freedom. Is it likewise in every park that is part of F3Nation? We imagine so. That is really why we do this, isn't it?

One day after soccer, Dredd was walking toward his minivan with his daughters when the youngest one asked him why there were never any police officers at Freedom Park. He had never thought about it until that moment, but she was right. Except at the front gate (enforcing the no-left turn rule), he had never seen a police officer patrolling the park. So he answered, "They are probably at other places where they are needed."

Which prompted her older sister (in her older sister voice) to say, "Yeah, we don't need them here because we have the daddies."

Little sister replied, "Rigggght, we have the daddies to keep us safe at Freedom. The police are at the parks without the daddies." At that, Dredd kind of looked away so his daughters wouldn't see the tears in his eyes, and he noticed that he could see about five other F3 guys within nine-iron distance, coaching soccer or cheering their kids on. And he knew there were another twenty F3 men that he couldn't see from where he was standing. But they were there.

It occurred to Dredd that if the bad guys came to Freedom they might have thought it easy pickings because they would see no police on duty. But they would be mistaken. If evil came to Freedom it would have the daddies to contend with, and it would not stand a chance. While we might be outnumbered, Brothers, we have locked our shields and will keep them locked in the heat of battle. We know that to be true.

Alone, we may go down fighting but we are still easily overcome. But we do not fight alone. We fight behind the Locked Shields of the Minivan Centurions. That shield wall will not be broken. That is Why We Are Here. We are F3.

ACKNOWLEDGMENTS

O UR GREATEST DEBT OF gratitude is owed to our wives — MDredd and MOBT – who have not only tolerated but actively supported our F3 passion and the related efforts it has spawned, including Men of Purpose and The Iron Project. If you found this book at all comprehensible, you can thank MOBT, who applied her editing pencil and sage judgment to this manuscript.

Gx and "Doc" Miller lit the fuse for the F3 revolution when they started the Campos workout at Charlotte's Freedom Park in February 2006; they later welcomed us into that group and supported our effort to plant what became F3 at A.G. Middle School on 1/1/11.

Every man who has ever accepted any position of responsibility in F3 – from Qing a workout to running the website – owns a piece of F3; in particular, we acknowledge the contributions of men who took early leadership roles in the Nation on the original "Q Board": Tango Delta, Girardi, Sweeper Boy, Haywood, Moniteur, Moses, Hyannis, Tiger Rag, Ben Franklin, Agony, Li'l Mike, and Smokey.

Our partners in the current Executive Group that oversees F3 Nation, AP and Crotch Rocket, deserve particular recognition. They have done more "on the ground" work than any other men in the Nation to ensure the ongoing growth and health of the F3 movement.

We've cited a number of writers, thinkers, and institutions that have shaped how we view F3 and its impact on the lives of men. As we've noted throughout, very little of the thinking we've done about F3, SadClown Syndrome, and the male condition in the early 21st century is original, so we owe a final tip of the cap to: Ori Brafman, Malcolm Gladwell, George W.S. Trow, the U.S. Army, Fred Borchelt.

Dredd and OBT
December 2013

ABOUT THE AUTHORS

DREDD (Dave Redding) currently practices law in Charlotte, N.C. From 1985 to 1994, he was an active-duty Army Infantry and Special Forces Officer. He is a graduate of the Army Airborne School, Ranger School, Special Forces Qualification Course, and SERE. He is also a graduate of French Commando School. He has a wonderful wife and three lovely daughters to keep his testosterone in check. In 2011, he helped start the men's workout and community leadership group known as F3. Since its modest founding in a grade school parking lot, F3 has expanded to a bunch of other parking lots. Dredd is currently the Nant'an of F3Nation.

OBT (Tim Whitmire) is a former journalist, primarily with The Associated Press, where he reported from Rhode Island, New York City, Kentucky, and North Carolina. In recent years, he has served in business development and executive roles for several firms in the middle-market finance space. He and Dredd started F3 in 2011; he currently serves as Chief Weasel Shaker for F3Nation. A native of California, he attended college at Harvard and is running marathons (or more) in every state. He, his wife, and three children live in Charlotte.